W9-CLM-350

HERE WE
GROW

WITHDRAWN

HERE WE GROW

Mindfulness Through Cancer and Beyond

Paige Davis

SHE WRITES PRESS

Copyright © 2018 by Paige Davis

All rights reserved. No part of this publication may be reproduced, distributed, or transmitted in any form or by any means, including photocopying, recording, digital scanning, or other electronic or mechanical methods, without the prior written permission of the publisher, except in the case of brief quotations embodied in critical reviews and certain other noncommercial uses permitted by copyright law. For permission requests, please address She Writes Press.

Published 2018
Printed in the United States of America

ISBN: 978-1-63152-381-6 paperback
ISBN: 978-1-63152-382-3 ebook

Library of Congress Control Number: 2017960220

For information, address:
She Writes Press
1563 Solano Ave #546
Berkeley, CA 94707

She Writes Press is a division of SparkPoint Studio, LLC.

All company and/or product names may be trade names, logos, trademarks, and/or registered trademarks and are the property of their respective owners.
Names and identifying characteristics have been changed to protect the privacy of certain individuals.

This book is a creative work based on my personal cancer journey, told the way I remember it. As I've learned from so many others, there is no one-size-fits-all when it comes to facing cancer or any other adversity. This story is a compilation of approaches that made sense for me.

For Aunt Sandy and Aunt Tricia. Thank you for your early illumination of this unimaginable road traveled. I felt your presence throughout, and you are in my heart forever. I miss you.

Contents

PART 2: BODY

PART 3: SPIRIT

Foreword
T. Flint Sparks,
PhD, former Clinical Psychologist and Zen Teacher

GOOD HEALTH IS NOT A "THING" you can have, like a new coat or even a friend, and illness is not the loss of good health that you must scramble to reclaim as if you have been tricked or robbed. Health and illness are one thing seen from different perspectives. They move together like waves on the ocean, surging and receding, informing and creating each other in every moment. They are two names for life, in human form.

What you are about to read is a personal account of one very special person's way of navigating the powerful currents of health and illness, and in particular, the tsunami called cancer that threatened to destroy her world. Like any life challenge, it is not just the details of what happened that tell Paige's true story, but how she responded to what happened, what she made of it all. How she was shaped and changed along the way, and, in return, how the world around her became shaped in response.

Life is always flowing fully, despite our opinions about it. Life was coursing not just through Paige's body—the "sick" one—but also through all of the intricately and delicately connected human hearts and minds who knew and loved her. A tumor was discovered in *her* body. *She* was given a frightening diagnosis, not me or you or her family members or friends. We all know that cancer is not contagious, but what we forget is that the feelings and reactions to the diagnosis and treatment *are* highly contagious. Everyone in this story had cancer. Everyone was affected by the disease and its consequences, impacted by the primal shock of what it means to be alive, and was asked to either face or turn away from this basic reality that was being revealed.

By entering Paige's story you also risk infection. You risk being changed. This is actually her invitation, her gift to us in the form of a potent, challenging question: "Are you waiting for a frightening diagnosis or other life circumstance to occur in order to live and love fully?"

This book is her response to her own question: "*Don't wait.*"

I was fortunate enough to meet Paige at the outset of her journey as she began to navigate her health/illness pilgrimage of transformation. We were brought together by Providence at just the right time. I've walked alongside thousands of people with cancer over the past forty years. Paige's clinical path from diagnosis through various treatment protocols was not uncommon. What was remarkable was her way of living through each challenge and triumph. She found a way to be alive in every moment without being trapped in the duality of health and illness. She was not defined by a cancer diagnosis and was not a "success" because she "beat" cancer. She was always herself, fully alive, finding her way with the help of everyone around her. I hope you will accept her invitation and follow her story of metamorphosis. In doing so, you have the opportunity to connect more completely with your own life force, and to wake up to the unstoppable and powerful vitality that runs through us all. This is the source of life. This is the source of real love.

Part 1:
MIND

"We delight in the beauty of the butterfly, but rarely admit the changes it has gone through to achieve that beauty."

—Maya Angelou

Prologue

EARLY ON A CRISP MORNING in February I arrived at our company headquarters, a cozy wood-frame house converted into office space, in Austin, Texas. The quaint vibe was idyllic for BlueAvocado, the start-up company I had co-founded with my sister and a good friend five years prior. Our company offers products like reusable shopping bags and storage solutions for people to live a greener, simpler life.

As I stepped onto the porch, I spied a beautiful yellow, blue, and red butterfly. It sat still on the railing, so peaceful. I craved that kind of ease in my busy, full life.

I watched the butterfly for a few moments. It was barely moving. *This can't be good*, I thought.

My co-worker Felix arrived. "What are we looking at?" he asked.

"A butterfly," I told him. "I think it's dead."

Felix peered closer. "It's not dead, Paige. It just emerged from the chrysalis. Its life is only beginning."

I once read that a butterfly "pops" its chrysalis by taking a deep breath. As I imagined the tiny creature before me breathing its way to life, I craved a deep breath of my own—*in and out*, followed by the wave of calm and peacefulness deep breathing brought.

Nine months earlier I had been on the verge of burnout, desperate for some peace. I manically googled retreats, spas, meditation, peace, burnout until I landed on a meditation retreat with Deepak Chopra, MD, at the Chopra Center in Southern California. Prior to attending the retreat, I was what would best be described as a "crisis meditator," tapping into the practice in desperation when I felt stressed or overwhelmed. My decision to attend the retreat seemed poorly timed given all of my other commitments, but I felt guided there, like I simply had to go. It didn't make sense logically or financially, but I'd never felt more at peace with a decision.

The first day of the retreat we were given a personalized mantra, a series of Sanskrit words, and told to meditate for twenty minutes by repeating the mantra. I needed more information. I needed to be guided. I needed someone to do it for me. But as I quickly learned, meditation and mindfulness isn't about creating moments of serenity, although that can happen. It's about meeting the moment at hand *exactly as it is,* with gentleness and non-judgment, despite how uncomfortable it feels.

That first twenty minutes, I must have peeked at the clock ten times to see how much time I had left. A million thoughts ran through my head: *I wonder what's for dinner. Am I doing it right? I suck at this. I can't do anything right. That's not a nice way to talk to myself.* I would catch myself and come back to the mantra, repeating it over and over in my mind. It felt like the longest twenty minutes of my life.

Over the remainder of the week sometimes the twenty minutes passed quickly and I'd feel peaceful. Other times I was restless, my mind dancing between my thoughts and the mantra. I learned that as we meditate we change the landscape of our brain so we become less reactive and more responsive, more connected to ourselves and others, and better able to trust our intuition.

In one of the question-and-answer sessions with Deepak, a cancer survivor expressed her frustration over not feeling peaceful and enlightened during meditation. What was she doing wrong? What could she do to improve her practice?

Deepak responded that all she had to do was recognize her thoughts of *doing* and *be* with them. *Do* and then *be*. "In other words, you *DO BE DO BE DO*," he said with a smirk. The modern day guru in his iconic glasses erupted into giggles.

Felix placed the butterfly on a leaf, out of harm's way. Like the mother of a newborn, I went outside every hour and checked on the creature. When I stepped out around lunchtime, it was gone. I felt bereft, and more than a little envious. I had all the makings of a fulfilled life—a successful business, an amazing family, a new boy-friend—yet I was miserable and feeling stuck in my life. I longed for something more, some deeper sense of meaning or connection. I'd been experiencing some tangible benefits of my meditation practice— I was sleeping better, feeling calmer in high-demand situations, and feeling more present in my life since the meditation retreat. Yet no amount of "do be doing" could deny it: I was jealous of the butterfly.

I wanted a new beginning, too.

Chapter 1:
The Lump

DAYS AFTER DISCOVERING THE BUTTERFLY, I have an appointment for my annual physical exam. I've been putting it off for months because of my work schedule. Meetings with investors, strategizing with vendors, and reviewing product development milestones take all my time, energy, and attention. I finally scheduled the appointment and am determined to keep it.

At the doctor's office I sit in a waiting room full of expectant moms and fill out the required paperwork. I've had three sinus infections in the last three months, and repeated cases of pink eye that took a month to finally heal. I attribute the illnesses to stress. I've also lost some weight. I assume this is a by-product of being in a new relationship.

The nurse leads me back and takes my vitals. When I step onto the scale, the number shocks me. I haven't seen those digits since high school. A jolt of pleasure shoots through me. I'm skinny. When my doctor comes into the exam room, we chat briefly about my life since I last saw her a year ago.

"Anything going on, or changes you've noticed with your body lately?" she asks as she begins the exam.

I hesitate for just a moment and then say, "I've had this pain in my left breast . . . it feels like there might be a lump there. And sometimes I can't catch my breath." A wave of panic floods me at this admission.

I've been keeping these symptoms at bay, refusing to acknowledge them even to myself.

The doctor presses her fingertips into my breast tissue. I wince as she probes the area I told her about. "How long has this been here?"

"I noticed the pain four months ago when I was getting a massage." I can't bring myself to tell her I felt it a year ago. A master at magical thinking, I had convinced myself it was nothing. My good friend and college roommate Courtney had recently been diagnosed with breast cancer. Surely the odds that we would both have it were next to impossible.

The doctor frowns. "It wasn't here at your last exam. See this dimpling," she points at the area around my nipple, "that's something we want to pay attention to. We should get you scheduled for a mammogram."

I can't get my head around her concern. I'm only thirty-eight years old. I try to recall the statistics on breast cancer. I'm pretty sure I've read one in eight women gets the disease.

I leave the doctor's office around 10:00 a.m. with an order for a mammogram. I freeze, unsure what to do next. I have a busy day planned but instead of driving to the office I head toward Whole Foods Market. I am suddenly craving a green juice, as if ingesting something healthy might somehow change my physical well-being in an instant. As I drive, I call to schedule my mammogram. The first available appointment is a week away.

I park the car, hang up the phone, and enter the appointment in my calendar. I move to open the car door but burst into tears instead. I cry the ugly kind of crying, the sort that verges on hysteria. I don't consider who might see me, or what they might think about a grown woman sobbing in the grocery store parking lot. I am too busy fighting off the fear.

I am the healthiest person I know. I'm dairy free. I haven't eaten red meat in over twenty years. I meditate thirty minutes a day, *every* day. I'm somewhat manic about it, which probably defeats the point, but whatever. I do yoga. Sure, I'm watching the clock most of the time and waiting for corpse pose at the end. And yes, I enjoy a drink a couple of nights a week and an occasional smoke with Herb Green, but all in all, I live a healthy lifestyle.

As we say in Texas though, this isn't my first rodeo when it comes to the Big C. My rather stereotypical Jewish family speaks only in code and in whispers about life-threating diseases. Saying the word aloud makes it real, and I'm not ready to do that yet. I've lost two of my aunts and three of my four grandparents to different forms of the Big C. My dad's cousin, who was like an uncle to me, died from it just six weeks ago. My heart pounds as I recall all of those funerals, all of those people who were so dear to me, all *gone.*

I need some perspective. I call my middle sister Missy. She and our eldest sister Megan are always the ones I call when I need a confidence boost. As the baby of the family, I avoid the pitfalls of competition or envy that define many sister relationships. They both adore me, and I look up to them. I'd moved to Austin to be closer to Missy and her husband Mark over ten years ago. She is my emergency contact in every sense of the word.

"Hi, want to meet for an early lunch?" Despite my growing fear I adopt a nonchalant tone.

"What's wrong?" Missy always knows when something is going on with me. I start crying again. Between sobs I explain that I have to get a mammogram.

"I'm coming with you," she says immediately. "It's gonna be OK."

In a small voice I hardly recognize as my own I say, "It's in a week. On Valentine's Day."

Chapter 2:
The Mammogram

I SPEND THE NIGHT BEFORE my appointment with my boy-friend, whom I've been seeing for about six months. I pick up Thai food from my favorite local spot and plan a cozy night at home. It's the day before Valentine's Day, and he arrives with a beautiful bouquet of flowers. I've told only my sisters and parents about my mammogram and wasn't planning to tell him, but I'm horrible at keeping a secret. As we enjoy our pad thai and a bottle of wine, I end up telling him about the lump, and that I'm having a mammogram tomorrow.

I'm not upset when I share the news. I am profoundly calm. I sense his fear but don't have the capacity to meet it. Our relationship is still very new. Dealing with the possibility of a life-threatening illness seems like an impossible reality. I assure him I'll be OK, and we enjoy our evening together with heightened tenderness, all too aware that tomorrow everything could change.

When the nurse calls my name for my mammogram the next morning, I hug Missy and walk back into the imaging room. The room is brightly lit, with pictures of cheery bright flowers on the white walls.

I change into a gown and head up to the mammogram platform.

The technician asks me which breast has the lump. We will start with that one.

She flattens my left DD breast into a pancake. It isn't pleasant, but I have a high tolerance for pain. She repeats the same process with the right breast.

"OK great, I think we got it," she says. "Stay here . . . I'll be right back."

I wait, literally twiddling my thumbs, for about fifteen minutes.

When she finally returns, the technician says, "I'm so sorry hon, we need another image of the left side."

After the second pancake flattening, she takes me to an internal waiting room. I watch as the technician consults with the doctor. Several other women who arrived about the same time I did are told they can get dressed and leave. I'm determined not to make much of it. I force myself to become engrossed in *General Hospital,* playing on the TV. It's been almost twenty years since I've seen the soap opera but Luke and Laura are still characters. They're having a reunion, and I quickly get caught up in their drama as if I've been watching daily.

Another nurse comes in. They'd like to take an ultrasound. I follow her into a dimly lit room that feels like my very own chrysalis, especially after she places a cozy blanket over me. Recalling the butterfly from a couple of weeks ago, I wonder if it felt a similar wave of uncertainty as it patiently waited to emerge.

The technician comes in, explains the ultrasound process, and performs the exam. I probably should be worried, but I'm too fascinated by the technician's ambidextrous skill as she manages the ultrasound wand with one hand and types on the keyboard with the other, all the while capturing various images of my breast. *Click, click, click.* She seems ultra focused.

The tech finishes and tells me to sit tight. "Can I get you anything?" she asks. *Wow,* I think, *they are really considerate here.* It feels as if I'm getting the VIP treatment.

When the tech returns, the doctor is with her. I know immediately that it's serious. I watch the grave expression on the doctor's face as she repeats the ultrasound.

"Is this cancer?" I blurt before I consider whether I really want to know.

"Due to the size and nature of the tumor, I do think this is cancer." Her eyes shine with empathy. "I'd like to perform a biopsy."

I can tell she feels horrible. In any other situation, she would likely just review the scans and call in the results without having to interact in this emotionally intimate way. But I've confronted her, and she's forced to answer. She shows me the healthy cells on the screen, and then areas of gray that are likely cancer.

A manic rush of thoughts floods my mind:

My cousin is getting married in six weeks. I bought a fabulous new dress. Will I get to wear it?

Will I have both boobs?

Will I have my hair?

A sharp needle prick brings me back into the moment as the nurse gives me a shot of lidocaine to numb my breast tissue. Tears well up and I'm sobbing again, the same way I did in the car in the Whole Foods Market parking lot. I lie on the exam table, sobbing into the deafening silence. The doctor lets my sister come in while we wait for the numbing agent to kick in.

Missy grabs my hand. "Oh sweetheart, you're going to be OK," she assures me. The blank look on her face tells me she is confused and shocked, too. I am not comfortable being the one in need of support. I want to comfort her. That is what I know how to do.

When it's time for the biopsy to begin, my sister leaves and my sobs subside. As the needle enters my breast, I close my eyes and focus on my breath, tracking it as it moves, *in and out, in and out.*

I flash on the meditation retreat. One of the facilitators had said that the true benefits of meditation like focus, connection, and presence start to show up beyond the seated meditations, in the times we don't even know we need them. I've meditated every day since that retreat. *Thank God for my practice*, I think as I continue to breathe. A sense of peacefulness moves through me. So much of life is outside of my control. Given my Type-A tendencies, this is difficult to grasp. Yet, because of my meditation practice, I am able to be in the moment, to stay present without getting caught up in fears about the future.

When the biopsy is over, I continue to follow my breath with my attention as I head back to the internal waiting room. I'm so glad to find my sister waiting for me. She has befriended a few of the women in the waiting room, and they all seem to understand what's going on. All of them look at me with compassion.

While I know the biopsy results need to confirm it, that's when it hits me: I have cancer.

My sister and I leave the office and walk out to the car. I feel a little wobbly, like I've had too much to drink. I'm about to open the car door when I stop dead in my tracks. I hear a faint yet clear whisper in my mind: *You've been in training for this your entire life. This is your moment.*

All of the personal growth and spiritual exploration I've undertaken in the previous twenty years swirls in my mind. I flash on snippets of memories: reading Bernie Siegel's *Love, Medicine and Miracles* at age thirteen, my psychic acupuncturist Nubby teaching me about chakras, Pilates training, the meditation retreat.

That still small voice is right. As if I am being shown the door out of the spiritual closet, I know cancer is going to be my most profound growth experience yet. It is time to open my transformation toolkit and get to work.

I feel giddy, inspired, excited, and relieved. This lightheartedness in the midst of such a dark hour is confusing. But I can't deny it; I am going to take on cancer through a spiritual lens that I have been crafting my entire life. It is as if all my curiosity around God, human-ity, and the universe is being crystallized into a force far greater than I can imagine. I feel enveloped in a vast universal love, what some people call grace.

Yes, I think, *this is who I am.*

Somehow I know that I will be guided each step of the way. I can't make sense of it, but it feels more real than anything I've ever known.

Then I get a text from my boyfriend. *How'd it go?*

Not good. It's cancer. Just like that, the lightheartedness disappears. I've said the word.

Now I've done it.

Now it is real.

Chapter 3:
Spiritual Flashback 1.0

I GREW UP JEWISH IN TULSA, Oklahoma. Besides my sisters and me, there were only five other Jewish kids in our school, two of whom were our cousins. While I appreciated the cultural aspects and family togetherness that Judaism offered, I didn't relate to the spiritual elements. I can barely recall the significance of my Torah portion at my Bat Mitzvah. My most vivid memories of that day center around the pink Laura Ashley sailor dress that I adored, and praying that I would not get an uncontrollable case of the temple giggles my sisters and I were notorious for.

I found my spiritual connection through Oprah. At age thirteen, I wasn't her target audience but I watched the *Oprah Winfrey Show* religiously every day after school. I related to Oprah's intrigue and line of questioning, intended to appease skeptics and call forth seekers. In college I scheduled my classes around the show, and at my first job I arranged alternative working hours. Anything for my spiritual fix.

Oprah's spiritual programming was sporadic at the time, but I soaked up the wisdom of Marianne Williamson, Deepak Chopra, Carolyn Myss, Christiane Northrup, Louise Hay, Wayne Dyer, and many other progressive spiritual teachers.

One day, Oprah's guest was Dr. Bernie Siegel. He had written a book about the power of the mind-body connection to heal diseases such as cancer. He believed that we all have a healer within, and that tools like visualization and talking to our bodies can have a profound positive impact on healing. He talked about a field of study called psychoneuroimmunology that identifies the connection between the mind, body, and spirit.

Then he said something I'll never forget: "Life is not a performance." Dr. Siegel explained that when you aren't true to yourself, your immune system gets confused. That's why people get sick. He was in the business of teaching peace of mind and helping people live authentically.

I was captivated. I needed to know more. I begged my mother to take me to the bookstore so I could buy his book with my allowance. While most girls my age were reading Judy Blume's *Are You There God? It's Me, Margaret*, I read *Love, Medicine, and Miracles*.

I revisited the book three years later around age sixteen, when my Aunt Sandy (my dad's brother's wife) was diagnosed with ovarian cancer. I spent a lot time with my aunt, uncle, and cousins who bookended me in age. Aunt Sandy and my mom alternated driving us all to tennis lessons, cheerleading practice, and Hebrew school. We ate Sunday dinner together every week, either at our grandparents' or at the Sleepy Hollow restaurant, notorious for its fried chicken, green beans, biscuits, and mashed potatoes.

Aunt Sandy's cancer is the first "bad thing" I remember happening in my sheltered childhood. The day I learned of her illness, she was having a hysterectomy. I insisted on going to the hospital with my parents and the rest of our extended family. About fifteen of us took over the waiting room at Hillcrest Hospital, the same hospital where I'd had my tonsils taken out just a few years prior. Aunt Sandy had brought me my favorite lemon custard ice cream from Baskin-Robbins.

The surgery took what seemed like hours. We kept busy, playing cards and eating snacks. It felt like just another family gathering, only it wasn't.

Ultimately we learned that the news wasn't good. Any time I was having a bad day, my parents would take me to the local Quick Trip for a Coolie, a drink akin to a Slurpee. The sweet treat always helped ease any pain or discomfort. When the doctor announced Aunt Sandy's prognosis, I did the only thing I knew to do, I ran out to the closest Quick Trip and got Coke and cherry swirl Coolies for the entire family.

A few days passed. No one told me much, but the adults' fear and uncertainty were palpable. I was an empathetic child, and I soaked up all their unspoken emotion with an overwhelming sense of helplessness. I had a strong urge to help my aunt get well. I returned to the bookstore and bought a second copy of *Love, Medicine, and Miracles* and gave it to Aunt Sandy. I don't know if she ever read that book or if it had any impact on her. I recall her telling me that it was challenging to concentrate while going through chemo. She seemed thankful when I gave it to her, and she was sweet to listen to me as I shared many of the ideas and techniques while we sat together in her study, where she rested after her chemo sessions.

Four years later, Sandy had held on as much as her body could handle. Like most of my family, I held out hope, but soon hospice was called in.

I was away from home, finishing my last semester of college in Indiana. On a gloomy February day my housemates wanted me to go hear a band with them. I'd been staying in a lot the past few weeks because I didn't want to miss a call about Aunt Sandy. My roommate, who was staying home to study for a mid-term, promised that if my family called she'd come get me. I reluctantly agreed and went out.

Someone pulled out a joint at the bar. I took a hit. I started feeling a little better. When the band came on, I quickly got lost in the tunes as I closed my eyes and moved to the beat. When I opened my eyes just a little, Aunt Sandy was hovering above the band. She wore a huge smile and was glowing. I thought I was tripping, and wondered what had been in that joint. A spark of light flew through the room, and a wind rushed just above my brow. I looked around to see if anyone else had seen the light. I was surprised to see my roommate standing in the doorway of the bar.

Dad had called.

Aunt Sandy had died.

Chapter 4:
Diagnosis

THE DAY FOLLOWING MY UNOFFICIAL diagnosis my sister and I had a conference call with the radiologist to get the biopsy results and the official diagnosis. We sat at Missy's dining room table and listened as the doctor rattled off cancer jargon and then explained its significance:

Ductile cancer (common);

Low/intermediate grade (good);

4.5cmm tumor size (not good);

Cancer not detectable in the one nodule they tested, but they needed to test more (neutral).

Treatment could include surgery, chemotherapy, radiation, and Tamoxifen—a pill I would need to take every day for the next five to ten years.

I was calm and focused during the call. I had two pages of questions gathered from my parents. (I had called the night before to give them the difficult news. They were steady and helpful.) At the end of the call the radiologist confirmed an appointment she had made for me with the surgeon.

"That was pretty positive," I enthusiastically told my sister.

"Sure." She looked dazed. I suspect that my eerily calm state freaked her out.

In that moment I understood something with certainty: my

sister and the rest of my family would be there every step of the way, but ultimately I was in it alone. I had no husband, no kids. Just Buck, my dog. The aloneness wasn't necessarily about a lack of people around me, but more of being alone in the spiritual sense; we come into this world alone and we exit alone. Ironically this awareness comforted me.

I was sure my parents were ready to take over. They knew what we were dealing with in a way I didn't yet comprehend. They had been through this already with my aunts, grandparents, and several friends. But moving back in with Mom and Dad in Oklahoma at thirty-eight years old so they could take care of me seemed more devastating than having a potentially terminal illness.

I sent a brief email to my family, summarizing what the radiologist had shared. I told them I wanted to take a few days before I discussed it further with anyone.

After a few days of processing my diagnosis in my journal, it was time to dust off my blog and reflect on recent events. I had started the *Sunshine Chronicles* about eight years ago in an effort to capture my insights about all things wellness, woo-woo, and sustainability-oriented. I wrote very sporadically, and had a loyal following of maybe five people.

It felt cathartic to be writing again. I also found the Bernie Siegel book on my bookshelf, and right next to it, my trusty copy of Louise Hay's *You Can Heal Your Life*. I'd been obsessed with this book in my twenties and still referred to it occasionally. It provides a comprehensive list of ailments, along with their emotional triggers and healing affirmations. I've learned over the years never to take anything— something I've read, an energy healing, etc.—as absolute truth, but merely as a perspective of my energy at that time. My job as a conscious, curious soul seeker is to be open to the lessons that are waiting to be revealed.

I had to get creative, but I merged the terms "cancer," "breast," and "left side" together and got the following: "Breast—Emotional Issue: A refusal to nourish the self. Overbearing attitudes."

"Breast Healing Mantra: I am important, I count. I now care for and nourish myself with love and with joy. I allow others the freedom to be who they are. We are all safe and free."

As I read this, it hit me—all of my seeking and living a healthy lifestyle had been coming from fear and angst to avoid the exact thing that was now happening. The diagnosis made me feel like I was being turned inside out. It was scary, and it made me feel vulnerable. I was skilled at shutting down emotionally and wasn't used to being seen by others in this uncertain state. Now I had the opportunity to approach healing with heartfelt awareness and expansiveness.

I took on cancer as if it was my latest business venture—strategy and tactical implementation merged with the profound state of vulnerability that I found myself in. I shared my plan for how I wanted to approach my treatment with my family in the only way I knew, through email.

Dear family,

I really appreciate your love and support over the last few days. It still seems surreal and I know the next couple of weeks will likely be overwhelming. I've set up my complementary healing plan and have some initial guidelines to share with everyone.

I get that this is my way of coping for now, and assure you I have had my breakdown moments and am not naïve to what lies ahead. But I also think that this is a crazy ironic blessing and I must be open to receiving the lessons it holds. I believe the plan below will help me (and all of us) to do this.

Welcome to Team Woo-Woo!

My Complementary/Woo-Woo Plan

Meditation - Thirty minutes at least once (ideally twice) a day.

Visualization - Daily, focusing on shrinking the mass.

Energy Work, Reflexology/Acupuncture – To keep my chi flowing before and after surgeries and treatments (weekly/every two weeks).

Talk Therapy - Weekly (1:1, group, etc. TBD).

Flowers - Fresh flowers (weekly).

Accessories - Stones, oils, house clearing, etc. (TBD based on need).

Nutrition - I have no idea what this looks like; I imagine getting pots and pans and learning to cook might be a good first step.

Team Woo-Woo Guidelines:

1. *This Is a Love Journey*—What's happening is shitty, but I prefer to stay away from terms such as "fight" and "battle," or referring to treatments as "poison." It is all healing energy, and this is a love journey that the universe has invited each of us on. Not to say we can't have some attitude—this cancer chose the wrong fucking body. My goal is to be as present as possible and to try not to get too far ahead of myself.

2. *Reach Out for Support*—Illness is often hardest on the caretakers. My cancer is as much a part of your journey as it is mine—I am just driving the bus. I need to know that everyone is taking care of themselves but realize I have to leave that up to each of you. Whatever feelings of fear, confusion, anger, or resentment are coming up, please seek support—ideally outside of the family. There are support groups for families of cancer patients, and I encourage you to explore those. At a minimum, reach out to friends when the situation starts to feel like too much.

3. Game Day Rituals—It is important to me that on the day of any meetings, treatments, or surgeries I feel as grounded as possible. I will visualize these experiences ahead of time and send light to the doctors, nurses, office staff, etc. At whatever level this resonates, I want to invite them to be part of the love journey. It is important that everyone feel the best they can on these days. That might mean dressing super comfy, or maybe in full-on glamour. Whatever the case, please treat yourself with love, empowerment, and compassion.

4. One Day at a Time—I am not naïve; this will be a long journey. I want to celebrate the milestones of every step. I'm not sure yet what that will look like, but I believe this will be helpful in staying present in the process of healing.

I love you all so much.

Here we grow ~ Paige

Looking back, I unintentionally set the tone for my healing journey through that email. I was trying to control *something,* since so much was out of my control. What the email didn't do, however, was give my family the time and space to process in their own way. While their responses were supportive and loving, mine was an approach no one had considered.

My family was accustomed to keeping news like this private and protecting others from feeling burdened. I had taken the pendulum to the opposite extreme. Expressing the emotive details of my journey was important for me, but what I lacked was the capacity to trust my family members to get in touch with their feelings on their own terms. Worrying and consoling others was my default mode, and I needed to offload that to make room for myself. My spin and tone on Team Woo-Woo was a clumsy, desperate, and lighthearted attempt to avoid the deep-seated fear we all felt. I was trying to fix for my family what I couldn't fix even for myself.

In hindsight, I might have changed the delivery to one of an invitation versus an assertive push, but the tools I wrote down came flowing from my years of spiritual exploration and experimentation and were exactly what I needed to hear. Even more important than the content was the simple act of expressing them. Writing became one of my most indispensible tools for processing my diagnosis and illness.

Chapter 5:
Spiritual Flashback 2.0

AFTER COLLEGE, I HAD MOVED to San Francisco and quickly immersed myself in all things spiritual, woo-woo, and wellness oriented. My friends and I spent our weekends exploring the metaphysical cornerstones of the city in the Haight-Ashbury and other historical areas. We checked out everything from crystal stores and psychic readings to Buddhist centers and astrology workshops.

One rainy Sunday we stumbled upon a cozy spiritual bookstore in the heart of the Haight. I was drawn to a bright colorful book with a rainbow heart on the cover. It was Louise Hay's *You Can Heal Your Life*. Her book became my bible as I preached the connection between emotional triggers and physical ailments to anyone who would listen. I quickly learned people didn't necessarily want their emotional issues scrutinized. But a few of my friends and family members were as passionate and intrigued as I was, and made me their go-to gal for all things woo-woo.

Aunt Tricia had been one of the first people to expose me to the metaphysical. When my Uncle Tim, who has always been an incredibly charismatic presence in my life, first introduced his wife to the family, there was no question that he had met a true life partner.

Born and raised in Montgomery, Alabama, Aunt Tricia had a strong Southern accent and nineteen eighties hair to match. I had never met an adult who was so fun to hang out with. Whenever she babysat, she shared stories of psychics she'd visited while we had a dance party to Aretha Franklin. It seemed we were always laughing.

Those fun times followed me into adulthood. When I was in my twenties, Aunt Tricia and Uncle Tim visited me in San Francisco. Aunt Tricia had developed her gift of photography in a more formal way and was starting a collection of capturing people's *tukhuses* (Yiddish for butt) to benefit a local organization. During their visit, Aunt Tricia ventured into downtown San Francisco and took pictures of a wide array of backsides. When we met for dinner in the evenings, she shared inspiring stories of the people she met, and I shared the new affirmations and the latest spiritual modalities I was exploring. Our times together were always filled with laughter and love. So much love.

A few months after Aunt Tricia and Uncle Tim visited me, my dad called me at the internet start-up where I worked. "Tricia is sick," he said. "It's multiple myeloma, a cancer formed by malignant plasma cells." I thought back to my sister's wedding a week earlier. Tricia had seemed fine. Before we said goodbye, Dad assured me everything was going to be OK. They were talking to the best doctors.

I froze after I hung up the phone. *This couldn't be happening.* We'd already lost Aunt Sandy. It had been over four years ago, but it felt like it had just happened. Tears sprang. I raced to the bathroom, where I cried out of sheer terror.

Was Aunt Tricia going to die?

What about my cousins, Steph and Ben? They were only twelve and fourteen years old.

I left work early and drove to Baker Beach, parked my car, and plopped myself down in the sand. It was a typical chilly spring day. As I gazed out at the vast ocean, the Golden Gate Bridge barely visible through the fog, I couldn't tell if I was shaking from the cold or the fear.

As Aunt Tricia started her various treatments, including chemotherapy and radiation, I grew desperate to share the many spiritual insights I was learning. I emailed Tricia tools I was sure would help her, such as making a photo album of the family and of her photography to remind her of the good times in her life, using particular crystals for blood flow and for protecting the heart, and reflexology and acupuncture. I wished I was there in person to help her. Sending suggestions via email was the best I could do.

Aunt Tricia replied to each of my "helpful hints" with an update on how she was feeling. She tried to maintain a positive attitude despite the physical challenges. She'd share news on the kids—Stephanie got her driver's permit, Ben was studying for his Bar Mitzvah. She also provided status updates on the influx of information I was sending her way. "Started making the photo album," she wrote one time. "The crystals are on my nightstand."

She always asked about my life, too. "How are you? Are you dating anyone? Are you writing? Keep writing. It's who you are." Tricia's encouragement about the short stories I drafted meant everything to me. She was one of the few people with whom it felt safe to share my writing. I had discovered my love of writing at age fourteen when I was away on a summer wilderness adventure. We were required to keep a journal as part of the four-week backpacking experience. As a result, I realized the power of words to express something deep inside. This passion sparked my studies in journalism, where I first explored writing short stories.

Around the time Aunt Tricia got sick, personal and professional stress were starting to get to me. I was having trouble sleeping and had chronic low back pain (both signs of not trusting the process of life, according to Louise Hay's book). I found an intuitive acupuncturist in Marin named Nubby. At the time I wasn't aware that he was intuitive (although I think most healers are), or even what that meant.

Every other Saturday I ventured over the Golden Gate Bridge to San Anselmo to receive treatments at the incense-infused clinic. As Nubby gently placed needles into my body to encourage the flow of *chi*, or life force, he taught me about chakras and energy through guided meditations. Nubby turned out to be my first official spiritual teacher. He profoundly impacted the way I experience healing.

"Imagine a grounding cord at the base of your spine. Feel that which no longer serves you flow through the cord. Let it go deep, deep into the earth. Now let the cord go," he encouraged as he gently laid his hands above my heart center. "Imagine your life force coming up through your chakras, the energy centers in your body. Imagine a rainbow of light flowing up through your spinal column; red at the base of your spine; orange below your belly button; yellow at your solar plexus; green at your heart center; blue at your throat; indigo at your third eye; white at your crown."

As Nubby guided me through these visualizations, energy flowed through my body. I left every session feeling peaceful, relaxed, supported, and safe.

Two years after Aunt Tricia's diagnosis, I delivered the eulogy at her funeral. I was devastated. That night I had a dream. In it Tricia said, "Come on, I need you to come with me." Together we flew around. Aunt Tricia said goodbye to everyone—I mean *everyone*—from family members to high school friends. It was swift and exhilarating. It reminded me of the time Aunt Sandy passed, except this time I could feel myself flying with Aunt Tricia in the dream. I woke abruptly. The experience had felt so real.

When I returned to San Francisco after the funeral, I shared the dream with Nubby, who explained that I'd been lucid dreaming, a type of dreaming in which you are aware you are dreaming. Flying dreams indicate that one is growing more in tune with a higher spiritual connection.

Something was being rooted in me during that profound time. I didn't know it then, but the words in those emails, the mind-body tools, and the spiritual insights I shared on Aunt Tricia's cancer journey would be the exact same ones I would later need and use for my own healing.

Chapter 6:
Cancerland

The Team Woo-Woo email spread like wildfire among extended family, friends, people in the community, and colleagues. It was overwhelming, but in a really supportive way. People shared heartfelt wishes and prayers. I hadn't posted anything on Facebook, but I suddenly received friend requests and messages from people I hadn't spoken to in twenty years—friends from camp, ex-boyfriends, even my high school nemesis. I felt like a celebrity, like I had hit the jackpot.

Only I hadn't.

I had cancer.

Regardless, I soaked up all the love and lightheartedness as I reconnected with many people.

At the same time I started the overwhelming process of navigating and scheduling doctor's appointments, MRIs, ultrasounds, and appointments for second opinions of all of these. As I looked at my calendar one day, I noticed an appointment that I had scheduled prior to the cancer diagnosis. Flint Sparks was a well-known psychotherapist and Zen Buddhist priest. When I'd heard him speak at an event years ago his message had resonated with me deeply. I'd been feeling stuck in my life when I had reached out to him three weeks ago. Our first appointment was coming up in just a few days.

Flint's East Austin office and Zen community center was in a wood frame house similar to BlueAvocado's. I immediately felt at peace when the gentle trickle of water running through a fountain and a statue of Buddha greeted me in front of Flint's office. When he opened the door, I was surprised by his tall, well-dressed appearance. He welcomed me warmly and asked if I would like any tea. I took a seat in the black leather lounge chair.

"What brings you here today?" Flint asked in a soothing, gentle voice. I was already feeling better. I proceeded to verbally vomit every detail of the past three weeks.

"Initially I reached out because I was feeling stuck. Then I found a lump. And then I got a mammogram. It's cancer. I've had two aunts die of cancer and my dad's cousin died just six weeks ago. When I was thirteen, I read a book called *Love, Medicine and Miracles* by Bernie Siegel, and—"

Flint stopped me. He asked me to take a deep breath. "I'm really sorry to hear of your diagnosis," he said. "I imagine this has been a very challenging time."

Tears filled my eyes. I'd been crying almost every day since that first episode in the Whole Foods Market parking lot.

Flint handed me a box of tissues. "One of my specialties is working with cancer patients, helping them cultivate their psycho-spiritual experience with it. I think I can provide some support for you." He goes on to explain that early in his career he became associated with an organization called the Cancer Counseling and Research Center that pioneered a successful model of emotional intervention and support based on the leadership of Dr. Carl Simonton. There he taught workshops, one of which Bernie Siegel attended and they made a nice connection. He later went on to consult in many cancer treatment centers across the United States including MD Anderson.

"Did you say you *know* Bernie Siegel?" I was like a love-struck teenager. I think it was less about Flint knowing Bernie personally and more about the validation that Siegel's work was real, and that Flint could help me. We talked for a little while longer about where

I was with creating a treatment team and protocol. I explained that a lot was still uncertain and that I was meeting with doctors and getting second opinions. We scheduled our next appointment for two weeks, when I hoped to have more information about my surgical and treatment plan.

"Once you have your plan in place, I promise you'll feel better," Flint said. "For many patients, managing the details to get a team and plan you feel good about is the most overwhelming part. Then we can start focusing on healing," he assured me.

I left his office with a sense of lightness. My team was starting to form—the right people and circumstances were showing up exactly as I needed them.

A few days after my appointment with Flint, I take my first step into Cancerland at MD Anderson Cancer Center in Houston. I have a vague recollection of visiting Aunt Tricia here years ago. It never occurred to me then that I would ever be back for my own health reasons. Staying true to my Team Woo-Woo guidelines, I am feeling cute, dressed in my boyfriend jeans, denim shirt with yellow sweater, maroon booties, and a navy blazer. I'm sporting our latest floral print BlueAvocado bag. It ties the entire outfit together. I look like I've stepped out of a J. Crew catalogue. I have a binder that includes insurance details, contact information, a living will, and a two-page bulleted list of questions, because that is the family I come from; we are organized and prepared.

A receptionist and a special volunteer host greet me and my family, all of whom have come along, and walk us to the Breast Center on the fifth floor. There are trams and restaurants, and lots of people with cancer walking around in a variety of scarves and hats, all available for purchase in the gift shop. I feel both overwhelmed and comforted.

The nurse calls my name, and my entourage and I head back. While we wait in the exam room, my dad pulls out a copy of the oncologist's resume. He reads her credentials aloud, noting that she attended the same college as my sister. They even graduated the same year.

"Let me see her picture," Missy interrupts. The look on her face is a combination of surprise and worry. "I think I know her."

"What!" I blurt. "What are you talking about? Were you friends? Please tell me you were nice to her."

"Of course I was nice to her. I mean . . . I honestly don't remember too much from college," she admits sheepishly.

Just as we are about to get into it, the door opens. The doctor looks at my sister. "Missy, no way! Oh my goodness. I saw the paperwork. You were listed as the emergency contact and I thought, surely this isn't the Missy I went to college with?"

They hug, and I breathe a sigh of relief thinking, *good one universe, good one.* I am starting to take mental note of these "coincidental" wins from the universe: butterfly, meditation retreat, books, Flint. Now the oncologist.

She introduces herself to my parents and then turns to me. "Hi, I'm Jennifer," she says with compassion and kindness. "I know this is an overwhelming time. How are you doing?"

"I'm OK." I try to stifle the cry that wants to burst out at her concern. She puts a hand on my shoulder, turns to the nurse and asks for a pen and paper. She draws a picture of what is going on with my cancer. I'm a visual learner, so this is amazing to me.

"You're estrogen and progesterone positive, and HER2 negative. As far as cancers go, this is a good kind to have. It is likely very treatable." That feels like good news.

"Your cancer is stage 2B. Your tumor is larger than average, which indicates surgery is likely sooner rather than later. This could mean a lumpectomy, or a single or double mastectomy. That will become clearer once you meet with the surgical oncologist. We don't have enough information yet to tell you the treatment protocol. I'd rather not jump to any conclusions and concern you with unknowns until we do some more tests." She explains chemotherapy, radiation, and Tamoxifen all as possible paths, but doesn't want to make any definite pronouncements yet.

Jennifer answers my entire bulleted list of questions—two full pages—with thoroughness and patience. She advises the nurse to make appointments with a specific surgical oncologist and plastic surgeon. I don't have to make those calls myself. That alone is huge. I love Cancerland.

The meeting with Jennifer is a huge departure from an appointment we had with a surgeon in Austin. My parents were biased toward me receiving treatment at MD Anderson since it is a Center of Excellence and both of my aunts had been treated there. But, it felt important to consider all my options, including meeting with the surgeon whom the radiologist had recommended. Unfortunately the Austin surgeon had been direct, harsh, and had a questionable bedside manner, a personality that didn't sit well with me or my family, especially my dad. After she ran briskly through all the treatment modalities and recommended surgery immediately, Dad spoke up.

"We'd like to get a second opinion. We have a family history with MD Anderson and you're our first meeting, so we need some time to process." His tone sounded aggressive and his nostrils flared as his papa bear protective nature kicked in.

The surgeon grew defensive in return. "You can do whatever you want."

I'd left that meeting feeling torn between the surgeon and my family. We'd started toward the car, feeling defeated. Then my phone rang.

"Paige, this is Melanie from the Breast Center at MD Anderson. We have you scheduled for this coming Monday at 9:00 a.m."

It had felt like another confirmation from the universe that MD

Anderson was the right place. Now that I'm here and have met Jennifer, I'm convinced.

My parents and my sister leave the room and Jennifer starts the exam. She examines my breasts and explains to me exactly where the tumor is as she touches my left breast. After I get up, she puts her hand on my shoulder again. "You're in good hands here. These are some of the best surgeons in the world. I'll be with you every step of the way."

Tears come as I choke out a thank you.

The next couple of days are busy as I meet with my surgical oncologist and undergo more tests, including additional biopsies, MRIs, and ultrasounds. I also meet with the genetic counselor and learn that I do not have the BRCA gene for breast and ovarian cancer. It's exhausting but I feel relieved to have everything under one roof. As we sit in one of the many waiting areas, I'm struck by the level of humanity that exists around me—cancer does not discriminate. I see so many people of different ethnic backgrounds, gender, and age. I imagine the various spiritual disciplines of these individuals and the familial and socioeconomic situations they find themselves in. It hits me how fortunate I am to have a supportive family and a strong spiritual foundation. I know this is not the case for everyone, and a combination of guilt and compassion fills my heart.

On our last day at MD Anderson, we have an appointment with the plastic surgeon. By then the surgical oncologist has confirmed that a lumpectomy is not an option due to the size of the tumor. I'll be having either a single or a double mastectomy.

When the nurse calls my name, my mom and I head back to the exam room. MD Anderson is a teaching hospital so it's common for fellows to perform the pre-exam. As I remove my robe and expose my DD breasts, the fellow says in a surprised tone, "Oh, yeah, we aren't going to be able to match those up." I smile, feeling awkward at his attention to my chest.

The plastic surgeon comes in. She is pretty, upbeat, and focused. "Hi, I'm Melissa. I'll be with you until the very end of this process."

I make a mental note for my universal "win" list—plastic surgeon with same name as sister.

Melissa explains that breasts as large as mine are challenging to match with reconstruction. "We can make them sisters, but not necessarily twins," she jokes to lighten the mood. Because of the size factor and my young age, she recommends a double mastectomy. The tumor is right at my nipple so they'll have to remove the nipples as well.

In the midst of making so many life-altering decisions about my health and my body, I feel grateful to have a decision made for me. I know it's the right one. Not strictly because of cosmetic reasons, but because I'm thirty-eight years old and I need to consider the statistics on how to best prevent a relapse, which is reduced significantly with the double. It is one of so many humbling moments where my vanity takes a back seat to the reality of the disease.

As we head to the airport, I feel exhausted yet empowered. I love how all my doctors insist that I call them by their first names. I trust Jennifer, the oncologist and team lead; Abigail, the surgical oncologist who will cut the tumor out and determine if the cancer has spread; and Melissa, the plastic surgeon who will put me back together. I feel comforted; cancer is what they do all day, every day. So much is uncertain, but I've found my oncological home at MD Anderson.

As I board the plane, my phone rings. It is the scheduler. Surgery is set for March 28, three weeks away. On the plane back to Austin, I start thinking about my Team Woo-Woo list and something that I can start doing now to prepare for surgery—visualization.

I recall some recommendations in the Bernie Siegel book and decide to have a "talk" with the cancer. When I close my eyes, I'm surprised by how quickly images appear in my mind. A cartoon-like cancer foreman shows up dressed like a construction worker. There are lots of other construction workers surrounding him, waiting for instructions. He looks me up and down and doesn't say anything, just smiles. He blows his whistle and calls off about half of his workers. "Let's go guys; this isn't as big of a job as we thought." He lets me know he is just leaving a small maintenance crew, tips his hat and wishes me luck.

Chapter 7:
Preparing

BECAUSE I AM OF CHILDBEARING AGE, I have to deal with the additional issue of fertility. Getting married and having children was something I always thought I would do, but somewhere along the way I'd convinced myself I didn't need a man to be successful and happy. I had been dating unsuccessfully for years. For a long time I thought love was something to do, prove, execute, owe.

Over the years, I started to develop the deeper level of intimacy I desired in relationships, including in the budding romance with my current boyfriend. While my diagnosis seems an unfortunate hurdle in the courtship process, he makes it clear that my illness doesn't change the way he feels about me. Whether our relationship is strong enough to sustain us is yet to be seen, but his support means everything to me. Still, this has little bearing on my current situation. I am thirty-eight years old, single, and childless, with a cancer diagnosis.

A friend pulls some strings to get me into the premier fertility specialist in Austin. I should be grateful, but instead I feel like a failure as I walk into the clinic. I'm humiliated, bitter, and resentful of all the eager expecting couples in the waiting room. I want to crawl into a corner with my cancer and call it a day.

The doctor steps into his office, where I'm waiting with Missy. An older gentleman with gray hair and bloodshot eyes, he looks distracted as he sits down behind an imposing oak desk and reviews my paperwork.

"So what brings you in?"

Seriously? You have the paperwork right in front of you. You know why I'm here. I have cancer, no husband, and probably no eggs, but everyone and their mother (literally) told me I needed to meet with you. So here I fucking am.

"I've recently been diagnosed with breast cancer. Given my age, my oncologist recommended I explore my fertility options." I hide all the rage that's simmering inside of me and play the part of the polite patient.

"How old are you?" He makes a not-so-subtle "yikes" face when I tell him I'm thirty-eight. "Fertility starts to decline significantly in your thirties, especially after thirty-five. Do you have a husband or boyfriend?"

Same "yikes" face when I answer a boyfriend, but not one serious enough to have a child with in the next week.

He launches into an overview of the process. "First we need to test your levels. Assuming they're good, we'll put you on hormones that could escalate your cancer since you're estrogen and progesterone positive. Next, we retrieve the eggs. We'll need to postpone your breast surgery to stay on schedule. Your eggs will stay frozen until you're ready for the next step. Once you find sperm, either through an anonymous donor or a boyfriend, we'll create the embryo and freeze that until you find a surrogate."

"Why a surrogate?" I hadn't considered that option before.

"Your oncologist will likely have you take Tamoxifen for the next five to ten years. It causes birth defects, and by the time you get done, you'll be forty-eight." Yikes face.

"While there is hope, it's a long road with slim possibility. I'm sorry." Finally, the sympathy I've wanted desperately since he walked in the door. I realize the "yikes" face wasn't coming from him. It was my own judgment toward myself. With each statement about my age and the truth of my situation, I feel like a failure at womanhood.

"I can send in the financial aid specialist," he offers. "She can walk you through the options. Good luck." He stands and reaches out to shake my hand. I feel horrible that I've been so mean to him in my mind. It's not his fault I'm without husband or child. I'm having a serious case of poor me.

I go through the motions of speaking with the financial aid specialist and take the blood test to check my hormone levels, but my decision is already made.

I call Mom on the way home.

"How'd it go?" she asks.

"It's too much, Mom. Even if I have eggs, I need sperm. Then an embryo. And I'd have to find a surrogate. Not to mention that the hormones will likely escalate the cancer. It's too much pressure for my poor little eggs. The whole process feels bleak and manufactured. I need to get the cancer out. I can't delay the surgery. I just can't." I start crying out of sheer defeat.

"Oh, sweetheart, I know how difficult this is for you. Whatever you feel is best, we support your decision." She makes me feel like it is going to be OK. But it's not. I know I'm making an urgent decision that will impact the rest of my life. I feel like I'm disappointing my family and depriving them of future progeny. Who am I kidding? I'm disappointing myself. Just like that, as I drive down Mopac Highway on a rainy Monday afternoon, I make the decision: No biological children for me. I try to gather my breath as I have grown accustomed to doing in moments of surrender. Like a trusty sidekick, it moves, *in and out. In and out.* Life is taking me in a different direction than I had expected or hoped for. Reluctantly, I try to embrace that.

While the possibility of having a family through other means is still there, grief over my biological childlessness continues to plague me. It's haunting at times. I don't hold any regrets but feelings of inestimable loss, sadness, and vulnerability still arise. I love kids—especially babies. In fact, I've earned the title of baby whisperer. I am beyond blessed to be an auntie to many, especially to my nephew Eli and my niece Ruby. I feel a love for these kids that is beyond words, and I deeply treasure my relationship with them.

I always hear new parents say how they never knew love could be so powerful before they had kids. While I can imagine it, and I have a sense this is what I feel with Eli and Ruby, I will never know *that* feeling. In this humbled moment I'm struck by the realization that the love I so deeply desire will never be based on something external— through a relationship or through having kids—but received by tapping into a reservoir of unconditional love for myself. I can barely fathom how to go about this, but I detect the faint whisper of the still small voice again: *You are loved.*

Chapter 8:
Let's Party

INSPIRED BY GODDESS RITUALS my friends and I practiced in San Francisco, I channel my fertility frustration by throwing a party in honor of my boobs.

A bon voyage boobs party seems the perfect way to honor the fourth guideline in my Team Woo-Woo email: One day at a time. I need a distraction from the overwhelming heavy dose of reality of the past few weeks. I'm craving fun and lightheartedness.

I organize my "bye-bye boobs" party in the spirit of a wedding or a baby shower. My sister sends an email invite to my closest girlfriends who have been reaching out, asking if they could do anything. I remember feeling helpless when I heard about my family members' diagnoses, and more recently, my best friend Courtney's diagnosis. I'd sent care packages, but had felt a nagging sense that there must be something more I could do.

Most people are confused by the joyous tone of the invitation, but celebrating milestones is important for me. As an entrepreneur, I was always living in the future and skipping over the present, on to the next hurdle before honoring the wins. I want to eke out every ounce of joy and acknowledgment possible.

I wake up excited the morning of the brunch. I meditate, then hop out of bed. It's one of those quintessential spring days in Austin; seventy-five degrees and not a cloud in the sky. I run to Whole Foods

Market to pick up some goodies. I'm *not* crying this time; I'm smiling and excited. I pick up fixings for bagels and lox and a frittata casserole I pre-ordered.

When it's time to get dressed for the party I want to feel bright and cheery so I put on a white shirt with black polka dots and a bright green mini skirt. My hair is in a ponytail. I look like I'm thirteen years old, and note the irony that age thirteen was around the time I longed most for boobs. But there's no time for melancholy today. Today is about fun. I put on Aretha Franklin and get my house ready for my guests. My sister shows up with Bloody Mary fixings. She sets the fruit platter, bagels, breakfast tacos, and frittata out on the counter buffet-style.

When the doorbell rings, I'm giddy with anticipation. My friends Kelly, Jen, and Natalie are at the door, gifts in hand. Forced smiles cover their shock. They haven't seen me since the diagnosis, and I've lost more weight from the stress of the last three weeks.

"Hi. Let's celebrate those boobs!" Kelly breaks the ice as she makes her way inside with a big box.

"What's that?" I ask.

"We'll get to it later," Kelly demurs.

We chitchat as we sit around the food. No one asks for details on my diagnosis or treatment, and I'm grateful to hear about what's going in their lives instead of focusing on mine. More people arrive. I am so happy. This is exactly what my soul has been craving.

The doorbell rings again. I look around, confused, because everyone is here. When I open the door, my friend Katie is standing on the doorstep. She flew in from Atlanta. I'm completely taken aback. It feels wonderful to receive so much love and support. It's still foreign, but I savor it.

Everyone fills a plate with food and we circle around the living room coffee table. It's cozy and sweet. Once we're settled, someone asks how I'm doing. *Really* doing.

I consider for a moment. "I'm really grateful. It's been tough, but my family has been amazing." I look at my sister, squeeze her hand. "Having a plan is so helpful. I'm just trying to stay focused on the surgery. One step at a time."

I provide an overview of the recent weeks' events, highlighting my meeting with Flint and how he specializes in people with cancer and their psycho-spiritual journey.

"Amazing," they all say.

Kelly speaks up. "Let's open presents!" She hands me each present, noting what it is and who gave it to me, so I can send thank you cards. I get crystals, pajamas, special clearing sprays, cards, Whole Foods Market gift certificates, haikus. So many thoughtful gifts. I soak up every ounce of benevolence.

When it's time for Kelly's present, she opens the big box she brought in and pulls out a stack of light blue V neck T-shirts for everyone. They say, "Team Woo." Before my tears get the best of me, Kelly hands out the T-shirts and we all put them on and take a team picture. I feel so grateful, and then glance at the picture. While my smile is genuine, I look skinny and exhausted. I don't recognize myself. But I also see the support surrounding me with all my gifts in the background. For a moment I feel like the luckiest girl in the world.

I meet with Flint a few days later. He listens as I voice my regrets and fears from the fertility appointment. He invites me to meet the fear and regret without judgment and pay attention to where I'm holding it in my body. I note my heart, and he advises me to just breathe. *In and out. In and out.*

"I'd like a visualization that I can listen to before the surgery, in the spirit of Bernie Siegel and his work."

I share that it's important to me that my surgical team feel confident, relaxed, and happy. I want to feel enveloped in a bubble of love, light, and protection.

"I think I got it," he says with a slight smirk. Clearly this isn't his first visualization rodeo. He places my phone on his lap so he can record.

"Let's get started."

Take your time to settle and get comfortable. Take that turn inward that begins as in any meditation or prayer, with your breath.

You are opening to this healing chrysalis and healing force that envelops you and penetrates you.

Imagine yourself surrounded by the love and care of the healing energy of your family and friends, which never leaves you. Your medical team is wrapped in that same care and graceful blessing. Everyone is in the service of the healing energy of your own body emanating from the inside, and they meet in this beautiful way. Your medications are assisting you in not feeling too much discomfort. Your healing is very rapid. Your incisions heal beautifully. Your tissues settle down with ease.

You allow yourself to rest deeply, sleeping as much as you need, resting and not taking on any undue pressure, stress, problems, or responsibilities. You find you are pleasantly surprised that you can enjoy this downtime, that it is like a new world where you get to enjoy being blessedly quiet, and at ease, and peaceful. It is something new for you to discover. With that gentle, peaceful relaxation in the present moment, you are spared the discomfort of jumping into the future, jumping ahead, because you find yourself so at peace in the present. This is where healing takes place, this is where receiving the blessings is possible; in the present.

After taking this time and deep envelopment of love and

care from your friends and family and your medical team, come back into this present moment. Take a deeper breath and bring yourself back into the room. When you feel ready, you can flutter your eyes open, grateful for the time spent.

I listen to this meditation religiously every day, sometimes twice. It penetrates my body, mind, and spirit. Warmth spreads throughout me, almost as if the love and light is transmuting my cells.

I am already healing.

Chapter 9:
Oh Happy Day

FOUR DAYS BEFORE MY SURGERY, my cousin Stephanie gets married in Washington, D.C. A happy family event is just what I need. I feel grateful to still have all of my body parts going into it. It's yet another universal win.

I'm hanging out in the hotel hospitality room with my family when I get a text from my best friend, Courtney. She lives in D.C., and I'm excited to see her. I go down to meet her in the grand lobby of the hotel. She looks amazing in a wig and hat combo.

The last time I saw Courtney was a year and a half ago when she was in the midst of chemo. I had expected her to be frail and weak, but instead she took me to a hot yoga class. "Gotta move the chemo toxins through."

She was amazing and inspiring. We'd stayed up all night talking, laughing, and crying. It was just like in college, only instead of smoking pot before a Phish concert, we smoked in her living room to help ease the side effects of the chemo.

"Paginah," she yells from across the lobby. Ugh. I thought I'd left that nickname behind in college.

"Court!" I run to her and we hug. I start to cry.

"I know, I know," she says reassuringly.

"What should we do? My family of course is dying to see you. Oops, bad choice of words," I say. We laugh—cancer humor.

"I'd love to see them, but first things first. You need to see my boobs. It will make you feel better knowing what to expect. I know it's weird, but it was so helpful when other women did this for me. I'm not one hundred percent in love with mine . . . it's like I have two blocks of concrete on my chest, but whatever."

I laugh, so happy to be with her. I give her an update as we walk up to my room—surgery will determine the remainder of the treatment protocol. Fingers crossed that the cancer hasn't spread, they won't have to take out any lymph nodes, and I won't need chemo or radiation.

Before my hotel room door clicks shut behind us, Courtney strips off her shirt.

"Wow!" I giggle at her new perky and somewhat large breasts that frankly look AMAZING. She giggles, too. We are like two giddy schoolgirls. She's right, seeing hers is a comfort. I'd always wanted a breast reduction; in a roundabout way I'm getting my wish.

I notice a scar above her right collarbone. "What's that?"

"That's where my port was for the chemo. Ugh, I hated that thing. But don't worry, you won't need that."

She shares some post-surgery tips: get this pillow from Relax The Back, get safety pins to pin the drains (which are little balloon like plastic containers that catch the blood and ooze from the surgical site) and get some cozy button-up flannels; you won't be able to lift your arms for three weeks. We talk for a while longer before my mom texts me that it's time to get ready for the wedding.

I hug Courtney. "Thank you, you have no idea how much I needed this."

"Oh Paige, you have no idea how much I needed this, too," my dear friend says. "You've got this."

Stephanie's wedding is the most amazing and meaningful event I've ever attended. Granted I'm in a vulnerable state, but it's heartwarming to see my cousin stepping into her new life with such grace and authenticity. I'm so proud of her. The dinner and dancing that follow are fabulous. From the flowers to the band, I am in a pink-hued heaven. I'm obsessed with posing for pictures with everyone, both because I look so good and because of the uncertainty I face.

Around ten o'clock, the party is hitting full steam. I'm standing at the bar watching everyone dance and celebrate when my pink-hued bubble bursts. I'm overwhelmed by exhaustion as I recall my cancer, my upcoming surgery, Aunt Tricia, Aunt Sandy.

From across the room Missy sees me crying. She comes over to me.

"I have to go," I say in a panic. I'm sobbing hysterically but don't want to call attention and deter from the celebration. She needs to stay with my niece at the party, so scrambles and gets my brother-in-law and nephew, and they escort me out.

"I just need to go to bed. I'm so sorry. I'm so sorry," I keep repeating in between sobs. I hate that my eight-year old nephew is seeing me like this. He's an empathetic child, much like I was at his age. I don't want him to worry about me or take it on. I want to protect him but my emotions are on a course of their own. My brother-in-law, nephew and I board the bus. We're the only ones riding. My nephew grabs my hand. "It's gonna be OK, Popo," he tells me with a concern no small child should have to feel. He started calling me Popo with some of his first words he could put together as a baby. "It's gonna be OK."

The next morning there's a gospel brunch with some good ole' Southern soul food. I walk over from the hotel with my eldest sister Megan and her husband. The restaurant is dark and bluesy, perfect for those with wedding hangovers.

I'm nibbling on a biscuit when my cousin Wendy comes over to say goodbye. There are tears in her eyes, and soon enough in mine, too. I hug her tightly. I wonder if she's thinking of her mom, my Aunt Sandy. I recall Sandy's sweet disposition and see so much of her in Wendy and her kids. My cousin leaves, and I shudder as I try to stifle the tears that are scratching the surface. The joy and celebratory nature of the weekend is coming to a close.

My cancer journey is the next big item on the family to-do list. It's about to officially kick off with my bilateral mastectomy in less than ninety-six hours.

The gospel choir is in the throes of their first set, singing "Oh Happy Day," one of my favorite songs (the *Sister Act 2* version). *Good one universe, good one.* My family lines up as I make my way through the room, saying my goodbyes. Each person offers me prayers for my journey.

"You've got this," says Uncle Tim.

"I'll be praying for you," says our family friend, Sherry.

"You can do this," my Aunt Janie squeezes my hand.

"You're the strongest person I know," says one of Tricia's best friends.

"I love you so much," says my newlywed cousin Stephanie.

I'm overwhelmed. I feel the presence of loved ones who have passed, especially my aunts and my grandparents. It's as if every spiritual entity I have ever wondered about is ushering me forward with love, protection, light, and compassion, just like in Flint's visualization.

I make my way through all of the goodbyes and walk out of that darkened room into the light of day. A magical force of love, which I have never known before, forever shifts the lens from which I approach my cancer treatment. My mom is right behind me. I turn and she looks at me with awe.

"Whoa," she says, referring to the overwhelming presence of grace. "That was incredible."

The day before I head to Houston for the surgery, I schedule a photo shoot with my new friend Romy. It's the last thing I want to do, but I know it's an important step on my journey. All I know of Romy, whom I met just a few weeks after my diagnosis, is that she's a well-known and gifted photographer. She learned about my story through my friend Jen, who had passed along my Team Woo-Woo email.

Our first meeting is in her South Austin photography studio, a garage apartment located behind a car repair business. She shares how she's watched so many of her close friends and loved ones experience illness, and how she would love to document my journey. I'm honored, but have no idea what that means. Neither does she. I have a feeling it might involve being topless, which previously I would never have considered, but things are already starting to shift for me, and my inhibitions easily fall away.

The goal is no goal—a first for me. My main priority is to capture the essence of where I am in a given moment. We decide we'll mark the major milestones, starting with my bilateral mastectomy. We'll figure out the rest once my prognosis is clear.

I show up to the studio wearing my favorite jeans, a black tank top, and light makeup, not my usual camera-ready face. I'm tired and depleted. Romy senses my exhaustion and I relax. She asks me to take a seat on a silver stool in the middle of the studio as she tests the lighting. I tell her about my cousin's wedding and how I can't believe I'm leaving the next day for Houston. I feel numb.

After a few shots Romy asks if I'd be comfortable sitting on the floor for a few more shots. Romy holds the space with professionalism and silence, not trying to fill it with idle chitchat. I'm so at ease I forget she's taking my picture. She asks if I'd be comfortable taking off my tank top and lying on my side. "Don't worry, we'll keep it classy and subtle. You can cover your breasts with your hands."

I don't hesitate. I slip off my top and lie on the cool cement floor on my left side, my left arm extended to support my head as my right arm wraps around my body. My elbow cradles my right breast and my hand holds my left breast—the one with cancer. Romy gives me subtle cues to shift my gaze up, bring my hips forward, but for the most part I just hear the *click, click, click* of the camera. I put my tank top back on and we take a few more shots.

The shoot was like a moving meditation. I'm really glad I did it. I feel calm, peaceful. Ready for whatever lies ahead.

Chapter 10:
Surgery

Dear Boobs,

It feels like just yesterday I was praying for your existence. A late bloomer, I spent far too much of my teenage years fearful that you would never show up. Much to my surprise, the summer I was sixteen you bloomed in all your glory. I spent the next few years trying to minimize your existence, until college when I met a group of girls who ended up being my best friends and were equally well-endowed. There were eight of us and we were nicknamed "The Rack" by the boys. Ironic that two of us have fallen victim to The Big C.

As I became more comfortable with my body in my twenties, I enjoyed the sensual aspects of your existence. From Australia to Austin, we've had many meaningful, intimate adventures, which makes saying goodbye all the more difficult.

I do not define my womanhood by your existence, yet my body is very important to me. This is the biggest challenge of my life thus far: to accept myself, the challenging journey ahead, and the uncertain aftermath. What I know for sure is that I have confidence in my body and trust its wisdom. I am a combination of cells based on millions of years of evolution. My body knows how to heal with ease and grace. My greatest job will simply be to get out of the way and let it do its thing. I'm just sorry it will be at your expense.

I know you have been doing everything in your power to maintain health, and that the cancer cells posed a great challenge for you. I am grateful you have kept things as contained as possible. You are officially relieved of your duty.

As I celebrate the good times we shared, I also mourn the experiences we won't have, especially breastfeeding a child. But while I mourn the path not taken, I embrace infinite new possibilities, which I cannot yet imagine.

As we enter our final days together, I thank you and honor you. Please know that while I may be a perky C cup, I will never be the same without you. With love and great sadness, I let you go, sweet boobies.

~ Paige

The day before my surgery I arrive at the Rotary House at MD Anderson feeling peaceful and relaxed. In many ways, the drive to Houston from Austin represents some of my last moments of independence as I enter patient mode. I'm used to spending a good deal of time alone in my protective little bubble, but if there's anything that these last six weeks have taught me, it's that there is so much magic in the act of receiving.

I'm fortunate to have health insurance that covers MD Anderson. I also feel very fortunate because I am still receiving a salary and have savings set aside for a "rainy day." I'm pretty sure cancer counts. Not all cancer patients have the means for such a high level of care. I'm grateful that finances aren't an added stress.

The Rotary House is the only hotel directly connected to the hospital. It's prime real estate; reservations fill quickly. I've booked two adjoining rooms with a kitchenette. While the décor and vibe is far from luxurious, with muted tones and a plethora of wheelchairs lining the lobby, it is clean, reliable, and convenient.

The staff is especially gracious. I'm greeted by a bellman and am struck by his kindness and empathy. "We're going to take good care of you here," he says as he opens my car door. He unloads my big suitcase full of pajamas and fluffy socks, my Relax The Back pillow, and a few other smaller bags that hold my spiritual accoutrements (crystals, clearing sprays, aromatherapy oils) and the medical supplies the nurse advised I get ahead of time (special dressing and ointment for the incisions, latex gloves to change the drains, Dixie cups to drain the drains).

My parents and sisters are en route. My eldest sister Megan has dropped everything at my request. She lives in Arizona, and had planned to come to Austin and take care of me for the second week after surgery but in a last minute, emotional and overbearing request, I've asked her to come for the surgery, too. I want the whole family here. I'm not quite sure why I feel so strongly about it. We all tend to regress when we're together, but I have this utopian vision in my head of my last supper before surgery.

My boyfriend continues to be supportive, but it feels like too much pressure to have him here, so per my request he gives me space. A beautiful flower arrangement greets me in my room, with a note from him: "I'll be thinking of you. Xoxo."

At 6:00 p.m. we arrive at my favorite Houston restaurant. It's dimly lit, with modern décor and soft music playing in the background. The hostess seats us at a round table. I ask her to take a picture. She takes several because each shot has a huge orb of light in it. I recall aloud that orbs and flashes of light mean angels are around. Megan, the more pragmatic of us, says, "That's one possibility. The other is that her finger was over the flash." I erupt in a full-on fit of laughter that we all need. Whatever the explanation, I feel grateful as I look around the table. I'm surrounded by my people. A unique combination of tension and somberness fills the air. Conversation is forced as we eat our meal.

After we order dessert, Dad makes a point to assure all of us that tomorrow will go great. "You've exhibited tremendous strength and presence," he says to me.

"And you guys," he turns to my sisters, "your mother and I are so proud to see you supporting each other."

I want to correct him that I haven't done anything; they have dropped everything and put their lives on hold for me. I will be forever grateful. But the words don't come. Just tears and a shaky voice. "Thank you all, thank you. I literally could not have gotten to this point without you. I love you so much."

Mom chimes in. "We love you, sweetheart. Let's just keep praying it hasn't spread. No lymph nodes, no lymph nodes," she repeats, as if convincing herself.

I wake up the next morning around 3:00 a.m., two hours before I need to check in for surgery. I sit up in bed, spritz myself with my sage clearing spray, take hold of the rose quartz crystal my friend Janie gave me, and put on my headphones. I select Flint's visualization repeatedly for the next hour, followed by a period of sitting in silence, hyper-aware of my breath. *In and out. In and out.* I get up, go to the bathroom, brush my teeth (being sure not to swallow any water), take a shower and clean myself thoroughly, as instructed in my pre-op exam. After a last look at my boobs, I put on the cozy green zip-up hoodie my Aunt Janie gave me. I note the coincidence of the two Janies as part of my morning ritual and count it in my win column.

My parents knock on the door. I open it and smile. "I'm ready."

My sisters meet us at the skybridge to the hospital. Mom grabs my hand as we all walk over together.

I'm shocked by the hustle and bustle in Admitting at 5:00 a.m. It's so crowded we can barely find a place to sit. I get my bracelet and am told I'm in group B, and that only one person can accompany me.

When they call my group, I fight back tears as I give my dad and sisters hugs. Mom and I follow the herd of patients lining up in the hallway.

"Are *all* these people getting surgery?" Mom asks. I don't answer. I'm trying to stay in my bubble. If my sisters were with me, they would be making mooing sounds. I can't help but giggle at the thought.

We enter the surgery prep area and the nurse assigns each person their own corral where a gown, compression socks, blankets, and pillows await. I change and then sit on the bed. The nurse comes in to see if she can get me anything while we wait for the anesthesiologist. She hooks a vacuum-like contraption into a valve in my gown. When she turns it on, I'm enveloped in warm air. It's like a warm internal blanket. I'm in heaven. *So far so good.*

Two corrals down a young girl screams as she fights the needle for the relaxing agent, the first step of the anesthesia process. I feel badly for her and want to tell her to breathe—*in and out, in and out.*

Mom presses my phone and headphones into my hand. "Put these on, you shouldn't be hearing this."

I slip on my headphones and play my carefully selected playlist, the one I envision my doctors listening to during the surgery. "Lovely Day" by Bill Withers comes on. I close my eyes and listen to the irony of the lyrics. A few songs later ("Here Comes the Sun" by Nina Simone), my surgical oncologist, the plastic surgeon, and the anesthesiologist arrive. They all ask my name, medical record number, and the procedure I am having. I must repeat this about fifteen times. Finally I get the relaxing agent as they prepare to put my IV in.

Ahh, OK. It's gonna be OK. In and out, in and out, in and out.

The nurse places another blanket over me, and I am officially in my chrysalis as they wheel me away.

I wave goodbye to Mom with a smile.

I wake up in a hospital room. I'm confused. I see Mom. "How'd it go?"
I ask.

"Hi sweetheart. You did great."

"Did it spread?

"It did. They removed twenty-nine lymph nodes. But they think
they got it all," she says reassuringly.

"Oh no, oh no." I vaguely feel warm tears falling down my face. *In
and out, in and out, in and out.* I fall asleep again.

A couple of hours later I open my eyes a second time. I'm not
exactly sure where I am, but Megan is there. "What time is it?"

"Hey there!" Megan chirps. "It's about 7:00 p.m. Mom just stepped
out to get some food with Missy and Dad. She'll be right back. How's
your pain? We want to stay ahead of it." Megan is a bit of a know-it-all
when it comes to all things medical. She's never studied medicine,
but she has an incredible intuitive sense and is intrigued by bodily
processes.

The nurse comes in. She is bubbly, upbeat, and moving fast. "Hey
there, sleepy head, how you feel? Can you tell me your pain on a scale
of one to ten?" I'm admittedly not feeling a lot but tell her around a
seven, hearing my family mantra of *stay ahead of the pain* in my head.

"OK, let's get you some food and a pain pill."

Over the next hour I focus on my cherry Jell-O, saltine crackers,
and apple juice. I take a pain pill and fall asleep again. Around 3:00
a.m., I have to go to the bathroom. They must have taken out my
catheter. I can't fathom how to go about getting up. I feel helpless. I
hear that still small inner voice again, the one I heard in the car after
my diagnosis: *"Breathe, sweet girl. You're surrounded by love and light."*

As I try to process what I'm hearing, the night nurse comes in.
She helps me sit up on the edge of the bed. The reality of the previous
twelve hours is evident in every physical sensation of my body—tin-
gling, throbbing, dullness, numbness. I am sore, heavy, and can't move
on my own. The flow of my breath is choppier than I'm used to. This

panics me for a moment. My mind is telling my body to take smooth breaths. My body does the best it can, and a series of sighs come out. I recall visiting Aunt Tricia at MD Anderson many years ago, and how she used to sigh all the time. With the nurse's help, I make it to the bathroom.

Win, I think to myself.

The morning after the surgery, I wake up as I have every day for the past nine months and meditate. I can't sit up fully on my own, and my meditation is probably closer to two minutes than my regular twenty, but being in an awake state, focusing on my choppy breath, and gently repeating my mantra is a reassuring comfort I desperately need. It provides an element of normalcy during this very abnormal time of lying somewhat upright in a hospital room, having been recently dismembered. It enables me to process and be in a present, grounded state to receive the outcome of the surgery.

Melissa, my plastic surgeon, comes in for her daily rounds shortly after my meditation, accompanied by a group of students, all eager to take a look at the new girls in town. "Hey! How you feeling? You look great, alert and awake. Do you mind if we take a look?"

It's the first time I can bring myself to look down at my chest. She opens my gown, undoes what seems like miles of bandages from my torso and smiles the biggest smile I've ever seen. "Well *OK* then." She shoots her physician assistant a look of approval. I sense they want to give each other a high five. It seems even they are surprised and impressed with their work. My boobs were so big before the surgery that they had the ultimate canvas.

As the plastic surgeon takes a look at my new breasts with the expanders (saline "placeholders" until we know if I'm a candidate for implants), she reviews her C cup creations (350 cc units). She explains that it's rare to come out with breasts this size immediately after surgery. Most women have to be "expanded" with saline injections to stretch the skin for several weeks before receiving their implants. On the upside, I likely won't need to be expanded. I am smiling as I take in their excitement and want to laugh at their reactions, but even giggling hurts at this point.

"That feels like good news," I say in a raspy voice. I'm struck by a sense of pride in my body and spirit.

"Absolutely. Your incisions look great. Rest up and I'll see you in a few days." She places her hand on my shoulder with a compassionate look that tells me, *You've got this; we're in this together.*

As the surgeon and the students leave, I feel uplifted, proud of my body and of my spirit for recognizing that lighthearted moment in the midst of so much pain and discomfort. I want to give them a high five of their own for everything they've been through over the last twenty-four hours. *Good job, body and spirit. Go team.*

"*Rest sweet girl, rest,*" says the still small voice.

Part 2:
BODY

When a caterpillar is inside its chrysalis, it creates a new form and structure. Unable to move, it dissolves into an organic liquid matter and forms imaginal cells. These cells are initially regarded as threats and attack the caterpillar's immune system. But they persist, multiply, and connect with each other. The imaginal cells then form clusters and clumps, begin resonating at the same frequency, and passing information back and forth until they hit a tipping point. They act as a multi-cell organism embodying the seeds of future potential, which contain the blueprint of a flying creature.

"The Story of Imaginal Cells," Imaginal Labs.
http://imaginal-labs.com

Chapter 11:
Recovery

AFTER A FEW DAYS AT THE ROTARY HOUSE, I get approval to go home and begin the next phase of my recovery. It feels like I'm in somebody else's body as I treat my incisions and drains. I can sense the trauma my body has undergone and feel great compassion for its healing capacity. I take on a new appreciation for my body as I realize how hard it has been working on my behalf for my entire life.

My parents drive me back to Austin. The trip is bumpy and uncomfortable. I listen to my surgery playlist, putting Diana Ross's "Ain't No Mountain High Enough" on repeat. When we pull into my driveway, Buck is waiting for me in the window. I walk into my house, ecstatic at being surrounded by the creature comforts of my home. Mom instructs me to rest on the couch and hands me my favorite blanket and slippers, the ones that Courtney gave me. I haven't let go of them since the surgery. I gaze out at the sweet little rose bush outside my living room window as Buck rests gently on my lap. I take a picture and post it to Facebook.

"Home. Healing. Cozy."

The likes and comments come flooding in. They are sparks of love and light, illuminating my healing path.

The limits of my body are foreign to me. I'm forced to move slowly, and use precision in every movement. My mind grows frustrated, trying to push me back to my old ways of powering through, but my body calls the shots as it continually invites me to rest, be patient, and take it slow. My meditation practice reminds me to focus on the physical sensations of the pain and emotion versus creating a story around it—heaviness on my chest with each breath, sharp poking where the drains are located, tender rawness at the incision sight, the warmth of tears as they stream down my face, constriction in my throat when I feel frustrated. I breathe through each sensation. *In and out. In and out.*

Each breath, coupled with mindful awareness, infiltrates my nervous system, naturally calming and relaxing me, bringing me back to the present moment and inviting true healing to take place. It's a place of embodiment where my spirit can naturally settle in.

Each day brings more mobility. Soon I'm reading work emails again. I'm starting to remember there's a world outside of the cozy healing chrysalis of love, light, and gentleness surrounding me.

My friend Katie is getting married in a couple of days. I was supposed to be a bridesmaid, but cancer got greedy and took priority. The day before her wedding, I'm feeling especially frustrated. I'm grossed out by my drains, my hair is disgusting because I can only take sponge baths, and I'm starting to go a little stir crazy. *This can't be my life,* I think in a moment of defeat as I look in the mirror after my morning drain cleaning ritual.

Megan is staying with me. I come out from my room and abruptly announce, "I'm going to Katie's wedding."

In a moment of crisis-management 101, Megan, who runs her own business working with executives and companies in crisis, encourages me to take a seat on the couch. "Let me fix you some oatmeal. And let's maybe take another pain pill?" she strongly encourages.

I start crying. "I need to do this," I say between sobs. Megan assures me I don't need to prove anything to anyone and that Katie will understand. I just had major surgery ten days ago; no one is expecting the impossible.

"I'm not doing this for Katie. I'm doing this for *me*. I need to know that my life is more than this. I need to feel like something bigger matters. I need to know I can do this. I want to be there." I try to get the words out between uncontrollable sobs.

Megan knows there is no convincing me otherwise. She hugs me and moves into practical mode, helping me plan the day and find a dress I don't have to slip over my head (since I can't lift my arms) and that will hide my six drains.

We chart out my pain meds and wedding strategy. I call Katie and let her know that I want to be there, but don't think I can stay for the whole wedding and reception. I suggest that I come to the hotel while she is getting dressed and ride over to the venue with her and Kelly (my fellow bridesmaid, who wins MVP for picking up the bridesmaid slack). I'll sit in the back for the ceremony and then sneak out.

Katie is shocked and thrilled. "Absolutely. Whatever feels doable. Just you making the effort is the best wedding gift."

It takes me two hours to get dressed. I move slowly, and I have to rest in between steps. Bathe—rest. I try to flatiron my hair by keeping my elbows close to my side and bringing my head down to my hand since my arms won't extend further. I'm exhausted after—rest. Put on dress—rest. Put on makeup—ready to go.

Megan drops me off at the hotel. I convince her I can walk in on my own. Katie is there to greet me. She and Kelly are the first people outside of my family I've seen since my surgery. They think I look amazing. I sit on the hotel bed as Katie gets her hair and makeup done. She looks beautiful. I feel so happy for her. But my body is starting to talk to me. I have to ask for an additional pillow to prop me up.

The photographers arrive and start taking pictures. Katie insists I be in a few of them even though I'm not in a matching bridesmaid dress. I'm too exhausted to argue, and happy to be included.

We're waiting for the car when there is a small crisis with the bouquets. Kelly takes care of it. It's so nice to be involved in someone else's drama for a while.

Katie's dear friend Joey shows up in a vintage collector's model red BMW. As we walk outside, Joey tears up when he sees Katie round the corner. She is breathtaking. It takes everything in me to stay upright. Kelly instructs Joey to help Katie and I get into the car while she gets the flowers. We make our way into a back room at the wedding venue. I give Katie a hug and let her know I love her and am so proud of her. As the music starts, I slip out and find a seat in the back row close to the exit. I don't want to see anyone. I don't have it in me to make small talk. I sit down next to a couple who are friends of Katie's soon-to-be-husband, Bobby. We've met a few times. As I take a seat, the woman grabs my hand and says how happy she is to see me.

The ceremony is beautiful and quick. Thank goodness, because I am fading. As Katie and Bobby say their vows, Missy pulls up. I quietly sneak out. When I get in Missy's car, I'm crying from a combination of exhaustion and pride.

I did it, I did it.

Win.

Three weeks pass and I'm given the OK to drive and start physical rehabilitation. I decide to pick up my Pilates practice after a three-year hiatus. I was originally drawn to Pilates in my twenties to help ease the back pain I experienced from my daily two-hour commute to Silicon Valley. I connected to Pilates and its philosophy that the exercises are meant to strengthen and lengthen the muscles. The technique results in a more balanced approach to moving our bodies, where the bigger muscles and smaller muscles work together. It also soothes the nervous system.

After Tricia and my grandfather passed away within six months of one another when I was living in San Francisco, I was in a state of uncertainty. The start-up I worked for was shutting down, and the thought of reinventing myself seemed impossible. I had a strong urge to flee San Francisco, the city that had once offered me so much emotional and spiritual growth. My sister Missy and her husband were living in Austin, and it seemed like a temporary safe haven where I could figure out what was next. The only thing that remained consistent during that period was my Pilates practice. It was a healing modality that brought my mind, body, and spirit together in profound and embodied ways.

When I discovered that one of the premier Pilates master teachers lived in Austin and offered a training, I decided that I could continue my practice and justify it with a certification. In addition to the physical transformation that was taking place as I moved my body in new ways, I gained a comprehensive and practical understanding of how the body and mind work together.

Eventually a few years after living in Austin, I opened a studio with two business partners from my Pilates teacher training program. There I discovered my love of teaching and healing. I felt empowered as I witnessed my clients connect with their bodies in meaningful ways that provided both physical and emotional strength. It was a metaphorical and literal depiction of the connectedness and the shared vulnerability that we all experience as we face our struggles around self-love and acceptance. While I loved running a studio and teaching, after five years my entrepreneurial spirit kicked in and I was eager to start something new. That's when I started BlueAvocado.

Now here I am, six years after leaving the studio, returning to the practice because I know it will be a huge benefit. Some friends gave me gift certificates to a local Pilates studio for my bye-bye boobs party. I cash those in and start working with Stephanie, a trainer I've known for years.

When I show up at the studio, she gives me a gentle hug and we get to work. We start slow. As we move through the basic movements of pelvic tilts, my body tries to pick up exactly where it left off but I don't have any sensation under my arm on the left side and I become winded quickly. While it feels good to be moving, even the most basic exercises soon get the best of me. I feel like a baby, getting to know the subtle and deep movements for the first time. I feel grateful to be connecting with my body in this way and continue to hear its message to be patient and kind to myself. And to breathe, always to breathe. *In and out, in and out.*

Chapter 12:
Chemo

SOON IT'S TIME TO MEET with my oncologist and discuss next steps. Megan drives me to MD Anderson, where my parents meet us. It's an official tag team as Megan drops me off and leaves for the airport. She is ready to get home to Arizona, and I don't blame her. She's been a caretaker in every sense of the word—washing my hair, driving me to see friends, making daily trips to the grocery store, helping me treat my incisions with special ointment, and many other little tasks I couldn't do on my own.

Mom, Dad, and I eat dinner in the restaurant at the Rotary House and then settle in for an early night. I'm exhausted from the drive and nervous about tomorrow, when I will find out if I have to get chemo. I close my eyes and fall asleep.

The next morning my oncologist Jennifer walks into the exam room and says that although the surgeon feels confident they got all the cancer, the fact that it spread to the lymph nodes makes me a candidate for chemotherapy. Devastated, I start crying.

Jennifer places her hand on my shoulder. "I know this isn't the news you were hoping for. But chemotherapy has come such a long way in recent years."

It's as if she's reading my mind as I think about my aunts and remember how life-altering chemo was for them. I recall Aunt Tricia looking at herself in the mirror and being shocked by how skinny she was. She couldn't tie her drawstring sweatpants tight enough to stay up.

Jennifer explains the protocol: sixteen treatments in six months. A combination of Adriamycin, known as AC, which will be given every three weeks, and then twelve weeks of Taxol, given weekly. Both drugs are known to inhibit the growth of breast cancer. I'll take Tamoxifen, an estrogen suppresser (since that's what fed the tumor) for the next five to ten years.

Jennifer explains the side effects: hair loss, weight gain, weight loss, nausea, anemia, and a slew of other possible ailments. "My good friend and colleague Debra is one of the leading oncologists in Austin. I will coordinate directly with her, and we'll do all we can to keep this as manageable for your lifestyle as possible," she assures.

When we meet with the radiation oncologist a couple of days later, it's determined that I will not need radiation. The surgeon had removed over twenty-nine lymph nodes but because the cancer had only spread to a few, he felt confident that chemotherapy and Tamoxifen were sufficient.

I am relieved to not have to undergo radiation, and soon I come around to being mostly okay with having chemo. I did some research and became convinced by the statistics and the many success stories similar to my case. Witnessing Courtney come through chemo with such strength and grace also gave me the hope I needed. By the time we head back to Austin, I'm convinced chemo is going to be a piece of cake.

It feels good to be back in Flint's office. It's been over three weeks and I've had a bilateral mastectomy since I last saw him. He lets me know how wonderful I look.

"I feel like an embodied case study of the visualization you prepared for me," I joke. "My body was primed to have an optimal healing experience, and it has." We discuss the last few weeks, and I bring up a dream I had the day before I learned my destiny with chemo.

I dreamt I was in a room with Courtney's husband. Several terrorists injected us with drugs. I recalled hearing about a cream that would make us immune. I felt myself falling susceptible to the drugs, and then Courtney suddenly came in. She had the cream. She quickly placed the cream on her husband and me and told us to hurry, that it was time to go.

Next we were in a little café, one we'd gone to all the time in college. Courtney was running around all over the place, organizing and planning. Her husband calmly stood by, an assured smile on his face. I looked over and saw my dog Buck. I was confused but glad to see him. He looked so precious all cuddled up. Courtney told me again that it was time to go. I looked at her, confused, and said, "But what about Buck? Who's going to take care of him?"

She smiled and said, "I've got it, come with me. Our friend Dave is going to take care of him."

I was confused until I realized that in the midst of all this, Courtney was trying to set me up on a date. I went over to Dave and told him that if he called my sister, she would pick up Buck.

He said, "No problem," and then started sharing all of these stories from college. We laughed hysterically. Courtney pulled up in a car with her husband, opened the door, and said, "We have to go back, but it's going to be OK. We've got the cream."

"I like to interpret dreams from the perspective that everyone in them represents some aspect of yourself," Flint says after I finish telling him my dream. "If you think of it that way, your consciousness is creating a blueprint for the next phase of your journey.

"Your friend Courtney represents the mental part of yourself that is organized, prepared, strategic, and responsible," he explains. "You trust her because she's been through a similar journey and is a tremendous support to you, like your own guardian angel.

"Her husband represents that spiritual grounding and presence you have within. Never saying a word, always there with confidence and assuredness that things are happening exactly as they should.

"Buck represents your vulnerable side, making sure your emotional needs are being met.

"Dave represents the unforeseen gifts of mystery and joy that arise when you let yourself go.

"And the cream is your healing spirit, there to protect you and help you to evolve to a new place."

I am in awe at Flint's adept interpretation and at how overtly my spirit communicates with me.

Flint walks me through another visualization, this one for chemo. He honors the first bullet of my Team Woo-Woo email, that this is a love journey, and encourages me to see the chemo as a powerful friend fueled by love and light, doing what it needs to do and then gently leaving my system so new cells can emerge.

As I leave Flint's office, I know that my journey is not over, but I have the ultimate dream team within myself (and in all my family and friends) to get through whatever lies ahead.

Dear Chemo,

Oh goodness, I'm nervous just writing to you. I've heard so many things about you, many of them not so good. Of all the challenges on my journey thus far, I have the most fear about meeting you.

But a funny thing I have learned about fear is that if you meet it and just sit with it, it can often reveal the most poignant moment of surrender. A moment where we realize that it is our defenses or reactionary nature to a situation, person, or experience that are oftentimes our greatest enemy. We have a choice to release any preconceived notions and to jump into the unknown with love, grace, and a whole lot of faith as our guides.

And so with that acknowledgement, I have chosen to see you as a friend. A powerful friend, for sure. Our friendship will be collaborative; I see you as a protector, helping to clear my body of any harmful, wandering cells. Together we will cleanse my body and ultimately recover and heal fully.

I know in many ways you will be my greatest teacher, offering blessings over the course of these next six months—some of which will be quite difficult. But I am up for the challenge and I welcome you to my healing team. I know you bring many friends along the way to support the work you will be doing, and I welcome them as well. I choose to see myself as strong, tolerant, energized, beautiful, fit, lean, inspired, creative, and engaging with the situations and people I love in my life.

I will welcome the quiet moments of rest, introspection, and many other unforeseen opportunities to connect with my spirit on an entirely new level.

Thank you in advance for being there for me. I welcome you with ease, love and light.

Here we grow,

~ Paige

I decide to meet my fears of chemo with as much celebratory attitude as I can muster. My friend Kelly recommends we have a chemo kick-off party. It is less elaborate than my bye-bye boobs party, but we gather at my friend Maggie's house for a happy hour celebration. My mom is with me. She's going to accompany me to my first treatment the following day. Maggie has margaritas, chips and salsa, mixed nuts, and other happy hour nibbles. Kelly shows up with cake-pops decorated with pink bows, and the words "love" and "light." I'm touched both at the thoughtfulness of the designs and that she remembered that I love cake-pops. She is the most thoughtful gift giver I know.

Other friends arrive with more goodies, including marijuana

treats. My college friends got news of the party and arranged to have a special vaporizer delivered that day. It's a cleaner way to smoke the pot. Mom is not shocked. She reminds me how helpful it's been for her best friend, who is currently going through treatment. I'm so happy to be in a relaxed setting with friends who continually show up for me in ways I don't even know I need. A flurry of emotions floods through me as I ready myself to take on one of my greatest fears tomorrow: chemotherapy.

My fear is admittedly influenced by the movies. While I have vague recollections of the challenges that Aunt Sandy and Aunt Tricia faced while undergoing treatment, I have more vivid memories of Debra Winger in *Terms of Endearment*, Susan Sarandon in *Stepmom,* and Charlize Theron in *Sweet November,* all of them throwing up and broken down. I think it's the throwing up that I fear most. I hate throwing up.

I wake up early the next morning, listen to my chemo visualization, and then dress in a button-up pastel shirt and leggings. I cut my hair a few days ago as part of a three-step strategy to prepare for losing it, and I'm loving my new bob. My port, which was surgically placed a week ago, subtly protrudes just below my right collarbone. This is where the chemo will be inserted. I place the lidocaine cream carefully over the port with a Q-tip and then cover it with Saran wrap as instructed by the nurse. By the time I arrive, the port site should be numb enough so that I won't feel the needle.

I fix a light breakfast of oatmeal and toast so my stomach is properly coated. My BlueAvocado bag, which I packed the night before, is stocked with healthy snacks of popcorn and a turkey sandwich, hard lemon candies to override the metallic taste of the chemo, my favorite blanket, new headphones purchased special for the occasion with an

Amazon gift card given to me by my high school friends, my favorite water bottle, and my computer so I can watch movies. I'm ready to go. Mom and I arrive a few minutes early. We meet with Debra, my Austin oncologist, and her physician assistant Sara. They are both warm and welcoming. Debra compliments my outfit and gives me my chemo binder full of information about the medications and expected side effects. The nurse takes us back to the infusion area, a room with lots of natural light and cozy lounger chairs lined up in six rows. I ask if I can sit by the window. The nurse tells me that usually they like first timers up-front in case there's an allergic reaction and emergency, but she's happy to make an exception. I settle into the chair and wait while the nurse gathers the various medications. As she prepares to insert the needle into my port, my mom grabs my hand.

"Take a deep breath. In . . ." the nurse pokes. ". . . and out. All done." I'm surprised that I don't feel anything.

She talks me through the protocol. "First, I'm going to take some blood and make sure your numbers are good to tolerate the treatment. Then I'll give you some Benadryl to prevent any allergic reaction. This may make you a little sleepy. Then I'll give you a steroid, which will help to prevent the nausea from getting the best of you. It may hype you up. And finally, we'll start the AC treatment."

All of the bags of medication hang from the IV pole to my right. The AC is bright red and labeled with a big warning sign. I close my eyes, put on my headphones and listen to my chemo visualization as the chain of events occurs. I'm not feeling anything out of the ordinary. In fact, I'm pretty relaxed and surprised by how friendly everyone is. Volunteers offer foot massages and donuts. Having my mom by my side and people checking on me feels very nurturing. I'm kind of enjoying myself.

I must have dozed off for a little bit because before I know it, the nurse is telling me I'm all done. They are about to flush my port with saline, which I've been warned is what causes the metallic taste, so in a moment of panic I ask the nurse to wait while Mom grabs the lemon candies.

As the nurse flushes the port, she walks me through the next couple of days. Nausea and fatigue are likely to happen around day three. She advises me to keep taking the anti-nausea pills. I'm reminded of the family mantra, *Stay ahead of the pain, or in this case, the nausea.*

I'm actually feeling great as I leave after my treatment. This is the steroids talking. When they wear off, I'm likely to start feeling some of the effects. But for now, I'm hungry, energetic, and perhaps a bit manic.

Mom and I meet Missy for lunch. I feel like I'm in that "Can you hear me now?" cell phone commercial.

Can you feel it now?

I don't think so.

What about now?

Still feeling pretty good.

Now what are you feeling?

Maybe a little nauseous. I'll take a pill.

Do you feel it now?

I think I'm OK. Maybe a little tired.

This continues into the next day. I actually feel like I don't really need the anti-nausea pills so I back off of them.

That night, it hits me. I'm so nauseous I can't eat. I just want to go to bed.

The next morning (day three) I feel as if I've been hit by a bus. Mom brings me oatmeal. I can barely touch it. I just want to sleep but force myself to do some light TV binge watching—*Arrested Development* on Netflix. It's a good distraction as I move in and out of sleep. Around lunchtime, Mom brings me a turkey sandwich. I force myself to eat a few bites. She always makes the best sandwiches. I continue to doze. Every now and then I open my eyes and see Mom checking on me.

Around dinnertime she gently wakes me up. "Honey, do you want a little puff?" She brings me the vaporizer, which I prepared ahead of time. I take a few puffs. It helps.

I decide to move out to the living room. I'm craving mashed potatoes, the ones we had at Sleepy Hollow when I was a child during family dinners with my grandparents, cousins, and Aunt Sandy and Uncle Lee.

Mom whips up a non-dairy version made with almond milk. They are delicious and totally hit the spot. I go back to bed.

The next morning (day four) I'm not feeling as bad. I weigh myself on the scale in my closet. I panic at the number. The chemo is literally eating away at me. I come out of my room motivated to eat and tell Mom I think we should go out for breakfast tacos. I force myself to eat two. It's more than I've eaten in the last twenty-four hours. It's too much for my system and I feel even sicker. We head home. I'm frustrated and tired.

"I don't know if I can do this." I cry in Mom's arms. She holds me, not trying to convince me otherwise.

Later that evening, I start to come around. The nausea is subsiding; I'm tired but not bone weary, where I can barely move. Mom and I take Buck for a walk. I think the worst of this round is behind me. I reflect on how the nurse predicted the various days and their symptoms exactly.

We can do this. We can do this.

Yes we can, says the still small voice.

I'm not sure exactly when I started to hear the still small voice. I have a feeling it's been with me all along. I imagine it is my soul, speaking to me in the moments when I need reminding that I am not alone. It seems to show up in dire, brought-to-your-knees moments.

My grandfather's passing was one such event. I was living in San Francisco at the time. My grief was guttural. It had been building for some time, as I had never really processed the loss of my two aunts, Tricia six months earlier and Sandy four years prior.

Grandpa was a huge inspiration in many ways, but he was an especially inspiring writer. For my grandparents' fiftieth wedding anniversary party, my parents, aunts, and uncles created a program that included excerpts from some of Grandpa's love letters to my grandmother when he was in the war. His words are heartbreaking and breathtaking as so much uncertainty surrounded him at the time he wrote those letters, never sure if or when he would see my grandmother and their new baby (my father) again.

Grandpa and I started writing letters to one another when I went to college. We continued through the start of the dotcom boom days when email became the popular form of communication. When the boom went bust and his leukemia started to get the best of him, his letters to me lessened, but I continued writing to him. I needed to know I was being heard, that someone saw me. Those letters were the initial tools that connected me to my soul. When Grandpa died, it felt like a part of my soul went with him.

When I received the call from my dad that Grandpa had died, I literally dropped to my knees. I wasn't a practicing Jew, but I was desperate to connect with something. I found myself driving through the streets of San Francisco and ended up at a Chabad. It was early in the morning. I knew nothing about Chabad—a Jewish tradition with roots in the Hasidic movement—but no women were taking part in the service I stumbled into. Seeing my distress, the attendant let me stand in the doorway. In that awkward, somewhat unwelcoming place of worship, I experienced a glimpse of a deeper connection, of something bigger, an indescribable presence that I now know is grace. It didn't lessen the grief, but it provided a spark within the deepest part of my soul, that place where abiding love, faith, and the authentic essence of our truth converge. I suspect this was the first time I experienced that still small voice gently letting me know *You are not alone.*

Chapter 13:
Chemocation

THE UPSIDE TO CHEMO: it's very predictable. After two cycles of treatment, I'm able to anticipate my energy ups and downs. I'm surprised by the things I can and can't do. Suddenly coffee, a staple in my life, is repellant to me. For some reason reading a book is difficult. I recall Aunt Sandy saying the same thing. Instead, I listen to audio books.

I learn to succumb on day three and rarely leave my house. Even walking Buck is too much, so Missy, Mark, and the kids pick him up for a play date with their dog Henry, Buck's brother. Day three becomes a day to simply get through with my cozy robe, trusty slippers and blanket, vaporizer, *Friday Night Lights* binge watching on Netflix, and Mom's mashed potatoes. It's a day where I welcome surrender and how hard, scary, and unfair it all feels. I experience moments, which usually occur in the shower, where I am literally brought to my knees. I pray for the support and guidance I can't muster on my own.

Surrender is tricky, especially for a recovering "doer" like me. I always assumed that fears were obstacles to be faced head-on. This is great when it comes to physical activities like bungee jumping or sky-diving (not that I've done those things), but when it comes to feelings and situations with no tangible action to take, it's a harsh reminder that I can't control everything. As a result, the unforeseen forces of strength, grace, and resiliency inspire me to rise. It is in these moments I know that I'm not alone because the still small voice reminds me.

Sure enough, I survive day three. Like clockwork, my body starts to recover again. I'm more resilient on day four and able to resume my morning walks with Buck. The walks become validation that I'm stronger than I think.

On day five I am rewarded. In one of the most generous gestures I've ever experienced, my cousins arranged to have flowers delivered weekly throughout my treatment. They usually arrive on Mondays, which are always difficult days. Nothing like chemotherapy to give new meaning to the Monday blues. Everyone else is getting back to their lives, work, and responsibilities. I resume managing chemo.

Each floral delivery is accompanied by an inspirational quote that always seems to provide the perfect sentiment/inspiration/encouragement, such as, *"The way I see it, if you want the rainbow, you gotta put up with the rain."—Dolly Parton*

I keep all the cards pinned to a bulletin board in my home office so I see these seeds of inspiration every day. The weekly gift brightens my spirit. More importantly, it reminds me of the energetic safety net all my friends and loved ones have placed around me.

Each day I get better. I nourish my body with healthy foods like salads and juices. Just when I start to feel normal again, it's time for my next treatment. I appreciate this predictability and grow accustomed to the cadence of my chemo lifestyle. I start to realize the moments of being brave and strong exist on the same continuum of knowing when to surrender, just at opposite ends of the treatment cycle. I welcome every experience.

My hair falls out in very gentle and subtle ways. I see it in the shower, and several strands come loose when I run my fingers through my hair. My family mantra of *stay ahead of the pain* is now *stay ahead of the hair loss*. I'm more concerned with the mess of the hair loss than with the vanity repercussions. I almost wish it would start coming out in clumps so I can just shave it, but there's a small inkling of hope that maybe I'll be the miracle case of chemo and my hair actually won't fall out.

I find a wig shop covered by my insurance and go wig shopping with Mom and Kelly. I don't have the greatest attitude as we arrive. I'm tired and just want to get it over with. Mom and Kelly are high energy and appear to be having a ball. I suspect they're trying to keep my spirits up. I try to force myself to have fun as I see myself as a blonde and a redhead, but with each new wig I try on, it feels like I'm trying to be something I'm not. I don't recognize the reflection looking back at me. After trying on several wigs, I select one that Kelly and Mom feel strongly about—they love it and think it's the closest to my current hairstyle. I get home and shove the wig in the back of my closet.

When I wake up a few mornings later, my pillow is covered with hair. I have a satin pillowcase that a friend recommended for this exact reason, a more gentle foundation for the hair and my head.

It's time to shave. I call my hairstylist Kristin, who I've been going to for over five years. She fits me in immediately. I've had short hair before, so I don't have too much angst. This part of the journey is the most traumatic for many women, and I feel like something is wrong with me since I'm not feeling more emotional.

I pick Missy up and we go to the salon together. Kristin gives me a hug and we walk back to her station. There are a few other people in the area so Kristin asks if I want privacy.

I tell her I'm fine. "Let's just get it done."

Missy pulls up a chair alongside me. I close my eyes, feel the buzz of the electric razor, and am soothed by the lull of the vibration as I focus on my breath. *In and out, in and out.*

"OK, you ready?" Kristin turns the chair around so I face the mirror. I open my eyes. Tears well up. Aunt Sandy's reflection stares back at me.

"You look beautiful," I want to tell her. Then I realize it's me. I turn to Missy in awe. "All I see is Sandy. Do you see her?" I must sound desperate, and perhaps a little crazy.

Missy is looking at me with a sense of pride and astonishment, her eyes full of tears. "You look amazing. So strong and brave."

I thank Kristin for making the experience so meaningful. "I guess I won't be seeing you for a while," I joke. She smiles and lets me know she's there for me in whatever way I need.

When we walk outside, I ask Missy to take a picture. I look like Demi Moore in the movie *GI Jane* in my black long sleeve T-shirt and royal blue joggers. I text the picture to Mom, Dad, Megan, and Courtney with the caption, "Thank God I have a good shaped head. Love you." A wave of empowerment washes over me.

I'm a fucking badass.

Because I am in the upcycle of treatment, I decide I want to celebrate and meet Kelly for dinner. It's the height and heat of summertime in Texas, so I can't bring myself to wear the wig. I've been watching scarf videos religiously on YouTube and decide to give it a try. I'm wearing a bright yellow shirt peppered with colorful flowers and a red scarf. I have such a nice time catching up with Kelly. As we walk outside after dinner, the heat slams me and I whip off my scarf. I'm so hot my scalp feels like a fireball.

"Ahh. So much better."

Kelly stops dead in her tracks. I'd forgotten how shocking I must look at first glance. "You look amazing," she says. "I have to take a picture."

I'm caught off guard and laugh as she takes the picture. As I look at the image she captured, I don't recognize myself. I am surrounded by an aura of light and see a magical blend of joy, love, lightheartedness, and happiness pouring out of me. It's as if I'm seeing myself for the first time.

As I'm getting ready for bed that evening, I keep thinking about the photo. I look at myself in the mirror, trying to make sense of what I witnessed in the picture. As I stare at my reflection, I see a glimpse of the powerful force of my soul looking through my eyes. It exudes a purity and innocence I've never known in myself. It's as if all the struggles I've been through the past few months are crystallized in this one moment as I see myself with such clarity. It feels as though that still small voice is integrated, and I've been granted the capacity to see myself and my life through the spiritual lens and light that has been with me all along.

As comfortable as I am with my shaved head, I am also acutely aware that it calls attention to the fact that I have cancer, and am therefore susceptible to personal insecurities, fear of judgment, and labels from others. While I try to maintain as much normalcy in my life with work and my relationships, I know I look sick to others. I see it in sympathetic glances at the grocery store. I see it in the overcompensation from my co-workers who tell me, "don't worry about things, we'll take care of it; you just take care of yourself." The team seems to be running fine without me, which I know is a good thing. But I have lingering insecurities around my job, financial security, and the uncertainty of what waits for me on the other side of this journey.

I also notice it in my relationship with my boyfriend. He is supportive, gracious, and patient. He continues to make it clear that he cares about me. Unfortunately our relationship has taken a backseat as I find myself in an ongoing cycle of recovery and healing. I can't help feeling like a burden. It takes all my effort to physically get through the day-to-day in this new body that continues to feel foreign to me.

I officially retire my girlfriend duties and we shift into friendship, meeting for weekly lunches. He keeps assuring me that we just need to get through the chemo and then we can get back to where we were before all of this. I don't have the heart to tell him there is no going back for me. I'm changing, from the inside out. I don't even recognize the person I was anymore.

As my internal awareness grows, I find myself in the unknown territory of having to let go of my perceptions of myself. Apart from the personal judgment and labels that have given me a sense of identity in the past—girlfriend, career-driven entrepreneur, loyal friend, avid Pilates student—there's a very simple and pure space of myself that is unknown. Untethering myself from the roles that I've been convinced for so many years describe who I am is uncomfortable, scary, and makes me feel weak. I've always known myself to be a strong person, inside and out. In many ways I still am. But having cancer humbles me. I discover that strength is a force that isn't necessarily about powering through.

There's a Hebrew term, *hineni* (*he-nay-nee*), that means, "Here I am." The one word I retained from my Hebrew school education is a powerful one. This is what I believe true strength is, showing up regardless of how we see ourselves and letting ourselves simply be seen and expressed in the world, often in our most stripped down and vulnerable moments. This realization serves as a powerful spiritual touchstone, reminding me that grace is the vehicle to experience the profound soul love within myself.

It's time for photo shoot number two with Romy. I'm excited and put on makeup and even bring a few wardrobe changes. I'm wearing my boyfriend jeans again, and while we agreed to take shots in the same black tank top from my first shoot, I can't help but wear a bright long sleeved T-shirt with a kaleidoscope of colors on it. The T-shirt makes me so happy. I also bring a white T-shirt, to offer some contrast from the darkness of the first shoot.

As I walk into the studio, Romy greets me with enthusiasm. "Wow! You look gorgeous." It's the day after my chemo treatment, so I'm still hyped up from the steroids. The day three crash comes tomorrow, but for now, I'm excited for my close-up.

We mix it up a bit, and Romy says she wants to capture some shots outside. Then we repeat the scenes on the stool and on the floor. I share the insights, perspectives, and silly moments that have occurred since I last saw her. We laugh, and delight radiates through my whole body. When it comes time to lie on the floor, I slip off my tank top once again, but this time I start giggling. I don't know how to navigate my new body. I don't have any sensation in parts of the left side of my body or in my expanders, but I'm nervous they'll pop. Romy cues me where to hold and support myself. I'm grateful for the guidance as I fumble my way through the different positions. I'm surprised when she says we're done.

"That was so much fun!" As soon as I say it, I recall that moment of walking out to the car after my mammogram and feeling that odd sense of lightheartedness in the midst of what should have been the darkest time. I give Romy a hug and stop at Whole Foods Market for a green juice on my way home. It's the last one I'll be able to stomach until day seven.

Dear Body,

Yowza, we have been through the ringer.

I focused so much of the last few years of my life on the emotional and spiritual aspects of myself that I feel like I may have neglected you. But this bubble of time where we are focusing together with the mind and spirit in equal partnership has been a gift. We have been poked, prodded, pumped, pricked, and pulled yet we made it through. Through the pain, awkwardness, and newfound connectedness, I feel like I'm getting to know you for the first time.

I will continue to treat you with the utmost respect and love through the second half of this journey. I'll nourish you with the foods you crave and fuel you for the road ahead. Most importantly, I will continue to be open to the lessons you teach me, regardless of how difficult they may be.

Thanks to you, when I look in the mirror I see and feel innocence, confidence, strength, light, and beauty that I have never known before. It's either irony or the most precious gift from the universe that it took being stripped of so much (hair, boobs, etc.) to discover this. Either way, I'll take it.

With love and gratitude sweet body,

~ Paige

It's midsummer in Texas and miserably hot. While I'm craving a vacation, it's difficult given my weekly Taxol treatments. My friend Rachel comes for a visit. She is naïve to what July in Texas means and is convinced it will be a welcome change from the gloomy San Francisco summer months. Rachel and I have been travel buddies since our twenties, when we both lived in San Francisco. She was part of my goddess crew along with my friends Regan, Tina, and Jamie. We called ourselves the soul sisters, in every sense of the word.

In her early days as a travel writer, Rachel was assigned various destinations to visit. Until she met her husband, I was her plus-one on adventures. We've visited five-star resorts, budget roadside motels, and outdoor yurts. It's only fitting that Rachel is the one who takes me on my first "chemocation," a couple of days in the Texas hill country an hour outside of Austin.

Rachel swoops into Austin, so happy to see me. Rachel runs at a fast pace; she talks fast, moves quickly and her intellectual capacity is remarkable. We head to dinner and have a lovely meal catching up but her phone keeps ringing. She's mysteriously distracted throughout dinner and keeps apologizing but she needs to take a call outside. I'm confused but ignore it.

We finish dinner and head home. Rachel's phone rings again as I'm preparing for bed. She answers quickly and then hangs up. "Wait! Don't go to bed yet, I think I saw something outside."

"Rachel, what are you talking about?" She's kind of freaking me out. I head to the door and open it to show her it's probably nothing. I'm shocked to see our friend Regan, all the way from Boston, in the doorway. Tears spring. I'm so confused, trying to process how Regan is standing in front of me and how Rachel was able to keep a secret. We stay up most of the night catching up on their lives, their kids, and my cancer. We reminisce and giggle and it feels like nothing has changed.

The next morning we head to Whole Foods Market and I note how happy I am, such a far cry from my initial parking lot breakdown. We grab coffee, breakfast tacos, and some sparkling water for the road.

We arrive at the Texas hill country resort around noon, just in time for poolside lunch. This is the first time I've put on a bathing suit since my surgery. I'm thrilled that my breasts are small enough that I can actually wear a bikini. Even though these are my best friends and I know they won't judge, I'm insecure. I feel incomplete. I still have expanders, which don't feel like they belong on my body. I compensate by putting on a swim shirt, justifying it by recalling that chemo makes me more sensitive to the sun.

We are enjoying lunch, laughing and talking about everything except cancer. I feel so grateful. I even gain the confidence to take off my swim shirt and go in the water in my bikini. The water feels amazing on my body. I've grown so accustomed to simply surviving that I've forgotten what it's like to feel physical pleasure. I really let go as I swim. After a few laps I'm a new woman in a new body.

When I come up out of the water, Rachel and Regan are smiling at me. They must sense the pride I'm feeling. Regan subtly cues me to pull my bikini top down. In my fully embodied swim, it rode up, exposing my nipple-less interim, expander breasts. Because I don't have any sensation, I didn't notice. Before cancer, this would have created more humiliation than I could bear. Now I erupt into laughter and pull down my top as lightheartedness fills me.

When I drop Regan and Rachel off at the airport the next day, my stomach is sore from laughing so hard. I am floating on a cloud of gratitude, love, surprise, and laughter. It's just the boost I need to move into the chemo homestretch.

Chapter 14:
Chemo Homestretch

ONE OF THE SIDE EFFECTS OF TAXOL is neuropathy (numbness of the hands and feet), and I'm nervous that I'll get it. My cousin, an acupuncturist in Atlanta, has convinced me that acupuncture could help. I know from my work with Nubby in San Francisco that acupuncture encourages the flow of *chi* (life force energy) and can keep neuropathy at bay. Through a friend, I'm introduced to an acupuncturist named Melissa. I note the happy coincidence that I have come to expect in my cancer journey—my sister, plastic surgeon, and now acupuncturist, all have the same name.

Melissa is enthusiastic, compassionate, and clear on my treatment plan. She offers a special financial package so I can receive weekly sessions throughout my remaining three months of chemo. At each of our sessions, we talk about how I'm feeling. It always starts with my physical ailments (nauseous, tired, achy) and occasionally is accompanied by an emotional breakdown (I'm frustrated I'm not performing at my normal capacity at work, I'm not feeling motivated to see friends, I get irritated at little things).

Recently someone cut me off when I was driving. I uncharacteristically yelled, "Fuck you, I have cancer!" It's the rare case where I pull the cancer card and feel good about it. (The other time was while shopping at a popular athleisure store, when the bubbly sales assistant said she couldn't accommodate an exchange. When I explained I was undergoing chemo and had lost so much weight I needed a smaller size, she reluctantly agreed. "Well, I guess we can make this one time exception," she said, rolling her eyes.)

I lie down on the table and Melissa inserts needles at specific meridian points all over the right side of my body. Because I've had lymph nodes removed on my left side, things like taking my blood pressure, blood draws, and anything with a needle are prohibited on that side of my body for the rest of my life. A wave of warmth and relaxation wash over me. I'm back in my chrysalis of love, grace, and healing. For twenty minutes I feel my body and spirit integrate.

The effects of chemo are cumulative, so while the weekly treatments are not as harsh, it takes longer to recover between treatments and the side effects start to get the best of me. For the first time I feel like my body is breaking down. The irony is that simultaneously, BlueAvocado is blossoming. We launch a new product line with our celebrity partner and receive amazing PR, with a full spread in US Weekly. I even manage to make a twenty-four hour trip to Los Angeles for the launch event. I have to wear a mask and gloves on the plane to protect against germs. At the event, I'm surrounded by eco-savvy fashionista bloggers and influencers. I'm articulate and photogenic. I have no idea how I muster the stamina to make it through the event, but I do. I suspect it's the last bit of powering through I'm capable of.

When I return, I realize it was too much. The side effects escalate. The fatigue is overwhelming. My eyebrows and eyelashes fall out, which I find more alarming than losing the hair on my head. Despite the profound love I'm feeling for myself, when I look in the mirror, even I can see I'm sick. My spirit is doing the best it can, but it's tired, just like my body. Worst of all, my taste buds vacate the premises. I text Courtney.

There go the taste buds (along with quickly thinning eyebrows :-) At this point it's just kinda funny. Or not.

She texts back, *Nooooo. . . Fuck - I'm so sorry. You're so close. Please keep up your stamina. Love you so much.*

These texts serve as a lifeline in my final weeks of chemo. For the first time I'm finding little solace in support from others. My philosophy of one day at a time is now one moment at a time. My breath becomes choppy. I'm sighing all the time; my body needs more oxygen than my normal breathing pattern provides. When I cry, tears pour from my eyes like I'm a cartoon character because I don't have the protective layer of my eyelashes.

In one of my final day threes, I can't bring myself to get out of bed. Missy drops Buck off after a play date with a Slurpee in hand. Tears fall at the simple generosity of the gesture. I'm immediately reminded of Aunt Sandy. I take a sip, but the sugar is too much for my system. For the first time since I started chemo, I run to the bathroom and throw up. Just like in the movies.

I imagine the butterfly as it was about to emerge from its chrysalis. It can't be comfortable in such cramped quarters. I wonder if it felt as annoyed, frustrated, and pissed off as I do.

Dear Paige,

You have written several lovely letters to me, which I appreciate. However, as your body, I have a few things to say.

First of all, why the fuck did you wait so long? You felt that lump for months before you sought a doctor. I'm aware of all the excuses: "It's nothing; I'm traveling; so-and-so needs me; I'm just stressed; I'm on deadline; etc." All bullshit. You, of all people, who claim to have such a mind-body connection, should know better. I love you, but come on.

Second, I will admit you have demonstrated an uncanny ability to be present each step in this process. However, it's been really fucking hard. We have been taken to physical depths that no person should have to encounter. I too am grateful that your spirit is as strong as it is and hasn't gotten lost in those moments. You've been so brave, but can you please recognize that you are experiencing those moments?

Third, can you please cut us a fucking break? You keep trying to push the boundaries of what you think we "should" be doing, but can you please eliminate that word from your vocabulary and embrace that we are in a time warp where the only priority is to focus on feeling good, being surrounded by people you love and who love you, and putting energy into situations that light us up—period? Everything else will be there at the end of this or not, but it's out of your control, so please, lighten up on yourself for the love of God.

Finally, please promise to listen to me and pay attention; you are worth it. There's so much we've learned together over these last six months and I too am grateful. I've learned that we really are a team, along with your spirit. Together we will always be your greatest teachers and provide exactly what you need.

I love and respect you in such profound ways. And while I know my language is harsh and my tone is angry, I am so proud of you. You're taking each moment as a great lesson to be learned and soaking up all you can. This is a blessing. Keep your eye on the prize, sweet girl. I'm with you every step of the way.

By the way, can you please pass this "pay attention" message along to all of your family and friends? You'll be doing a huge favor for bodies everywhere.

- Your Body

p.s. Apologies for repetitive use of the word FUCK, but don't you just feel better when you say it?

Mom and Dad come in for my last chemo session. I've ordered cake-pops for the nurses as a thank you. After I complete my final infusion, I'm enthusiastically greeted by the nurses, doctors, and other patients. They shower me with confetti and grant me my certificate of chemo completion. I'm overwhelmed and in tears as usual. This community has nurtured me in a way that gives new meaning to the sentiment that it takes a village.

Finally it is my turn. I get to ring the bell, the one I've enviously watched so many others ring these last six months. Its ring reverberates joy, love, and light throughout my being. I'm done with chemo.

I can't believe I made it.

I fully appreciate the kaleidoscopic moments that mark my chemo journey. The moments where light and dark converged, reminding me that life is full of endings and beginnings, losses and love, fear and faith. I have no idea what lies ahead. While cancer hasn't defined me, it has transformed and transmuted me. I walk in the world with a new perspective and with a glimpse of a higher version of myself. The collective and collaborative energy from others is perhaps one of the most important gifts my journey through cancer has taught me; not only could I not do it on my own, *I'm not meant to.* It is our birthright as spiritual beings living this human experience to love and to be loved, to connect with others, and to show up, even when we don't know how to do so. I am proud and humbled.

But as I leave the infusion room for the last time, I can't help but think, *now what?*

Part 3:
SPIRIT

When the butterfly first emerges from the chrysalis, both of the wings are soft and folded against its body. The butterfly had to fit all its new parts inside the chrysalis. As soon as the butterfly has rested after coming out of the chrysalis, it pumps blood into its wings to get them working and flapping. Then it gets to fly.

"Butterfly Life Cycle / Butterfly Metamorphosis,"
The Butterfly Site. http://www.thebutterflysite.com

Chapter 15:
Survivor/Thriver

I POST MY BELL RINGING ON FACEBOOK.

We did it! I've got the confetti, diploma, and bell ringing to prove it. Thx for all the support and love. #12 of 12 - check! #seeyachemo

I am filled with gratitude by the congratulatory sentiments that pour in. Many of my friends and family have been on this journey with me, virtually and in person. This is as much their milestone as it is mine. People comment repeatedly about how amazed they've been by my positive attitude throughout treatment.

This confuses me, because I'm very aware of the hardship of this time. What others perceive as positive is really about being present. I know this is confusing to people. I too used to be skeptical of the notion of being present, especially during challenging moments.

But cancer and its trusty sidekick mortality have taught me a lot about presence. In many ways, it's the only option—the past is gone, the future is yet to happen. The present moment is all there is. The moment at hand always gives me what I need—my breath, feeling an emotion, or even experiencing my still small voice. Everything is amplified in this space—peace, sadness, joy—but all is met fully and creates the current of my life. It isn't about stagnation, but still-ness. Through stillness, I become enlivened and more mindful. It's like a muscle I flex through my meditation practice. It allows my body, mind, and spirit to connect so I'm able to respond versus react to whatever challenge or opportunity exists with greater connection, focus, discernment, and appreciation for the moment at hand.

Presence is the persistent invitation to release and surrender, realizing there is something bigger at play. It reminds me that without question, I'm part of a collective consciousness, interconnected to every living being, the cosmos, spirit, and, because I believe, even God.

I didn't arrive at this place of embracing present-moment awareness and letting go overnight. My ability to feel and emote throughout my journey is the result of years of dabbling in various spiritual modalities in an effort to gain insight into the bigger picture of myself and to make meaning of it all. Over the years, I slowly started to understand that emotion was the gateway to surrender. The old cliché "you gotta feel to heal" became a mantra in my unfolding spiritual awareness while I was still living in San Francisco, and took on a deeper significance when I pursued my Pilates certification after moving to Austin. During this period, I found myself in a wellness and personal growth community I never knew existed. It was a Mecca of modalities that provided new ways to connect with my spirit.

I encountered major spiritual breakthroughs through Holographic Repatterning, a process that works with the self-healing energy within the body-mind system. I became aware of the limiting beliefs that held me back in my relationships. I explored my Akashic records, an energetic imprint of every thought, action, emotion, and experience that has ever occurred in time and space. This is where I learned about past lives and other more "out-there" principles that strangely provided perspective on my life experiences. I received myofascial massage, a form of deep yet gentle physical therapy that releases the connective tissue surrounding our muscles and bones, where some of the deepest physical and emotional traumas become trapped. Some of it could be described as very woo-woo, but relevant and meaningful.

The thing I didn't fully comprehend when I began these deeply healing modalities but am now appreciating through my cancer journey was that it's not necessarily a "one and done." Initial sessions were often about identifying energetic, emotional, or physical blocks and bringing awareness and healing so they could be released. This breakdown process can be emotionally and physically painful. Tears upon tears are likely to follow, however not always immediately. I wasn't prepared for the waves of feelings that resulted from the work, which followed days, sometimes weeks, later. There was always a lightness of being that awaited as I consciously worked with the cathartic flow.

During this time of cathartic discovery, I learned to embrace the more difficult emotions such as fear, anger, and sadness as the breakdowns that always lead to *breakthroughs*. While some of my breakdowns have been heart-wrenching, they were due to the energetic density of years of stress, unrealistic and unrealized expectations, and holding onto outcomes that I had no control over. I've learned that so much of healing is simply about being aware of my actions and behaviors, and in most cases forgiving myself and others. Through this process, an expansiveness arises that serves as an invitation to live wholeheartedly.

I now realize in my post-chemo recovery that my body holds my stories. With love and acceptance I invite a level of transmutation where deep healing can take hold and I'm able to witness my spirit merging with my physicality. I feel myself becoming a more fully embodied version of myself and feel connected to my truth, light, and love that naturally come shining through.

I'm not sure exactly where on my path this connection first got lost. I suppose that it got dimmer and dimmer as life stressors and responsibilities got in the way. But I can see now that the moment of burnout that propelled me to attend that meditation retreat at the Chopra Center wasn't about my job or my relationships. It was about my disconnection from my spirit.

I knew from the moment I sent that first Team Woo-Woo email

that expressing my journey through writing would serve as a powerful healing modality to reunite with my spirit and the ultimate tool to bring me into this state of present-moment awareness. Writing became as important as the chemo, acupuncture, meditation, my sessions with Flint, and the many other tools of transformation I used and continue to tap into. It also served as a record of my experience so I could reflect on the many lessons learned and celebrate the successes, the "wins."

I look back at the first Facebook post after my surgery and feel proud that I was up and around after just one week. But I also recall the pain that kept me up at night, and the nauseating process of clearing my drains. I often cried myself to sleep, wondering how I would make it through. I can look at pictures of my sweet puppy Buck as a reflection of the joy that got me up in the morning. And while I embrace all of the amazing love and support of my many friends and family, most nights, it was just me. Sometimes that was really scary.

While I see vibrancy in my face in pictures of myself from that time, I don't recognize that version of me, a bald, browless, eyelashless, dry, sick person. This journey hasn't been about putting on a brave face. I have confronted my deepest fears. I've experienced moments of profound grace, love, faith, and self-compassion. I pray these moments become my mainstay, keeping me guided, focused, and connected to the deepest part of myself as I move forward.

The weeks following my graduation from chemo are a little bit confusing. Mentally I know I'm done, but physically I still feel crummy. I had this vision that the day after my last chemo treatment I would be ready to party and get going with my life again. While on one level I know that I am irrevocably changed, another part of me wants the change to be minimal and controllable. But these are unrealistic expectations.

Sure I have additional appointments, treatments, and surgeries ahead of me, but when I look at what I've just accomplished, I feel like a rock star. I thought my hair would grow out like a supercharged chia pet, and I would have my super cute pixie cut and fantastic brows and lashes back in a week. I thought I'd be inspired to write every day and engage with work with new enthusiasm. I thought I'd have the strength to get back to my hot yoga class. I thought I would have the energy to call and spend time with all the people I love who I hadn't been able to connect with the last several months.

Instead I feel more exhausted than ever. My body is still shedding its final course of chemo. I know the importance of continuing to nurture my body with what it desires in this new regeneration phase. I trust the guidance of my intuition and honor the voice within to guide me. I recall the words of Deepak Chopra. *Do be do be do* becomes my new mantra as I patiently discover a new cadence of emerging in the world and give my body the rest it still desperately needs.

I'm surprised by the loneliness I feel during the weeks following chemo. I expected to feel elated that treatment is over, but *everything* about treatment is over. The constant attention, and the chemo community I visited weekly that nurtured me. I'd grown accustomed to these things. Without them I feel disoriented. Despite being surrounded by love and support, I'm on my own, living the life of a survivor or thriver, as many people call it, uncertain what that means. I feel like the teacher in *Ferris Bueller's Day Off*—looking for someone, anyone, to tell me what I'm supposed to do next. But those answers have to come from me.

Meditation serves as my source of connection. I crave it even more as I find myself unsure what going forward looks like in my work, my personal life, and my physical being. I'm reminded of the morning after my surgery, and the importance of breathing consciously and repeating my mantra. During meditation I find myself practicing one of my favorite mindfulness techniques, paying attention to the natural pause that occurs between the inhale and the exhale. Physiologically I find it supportive in my slower pacing. No matter the length of the pause, it instills a trust that the next breath always arrives.

All of these feelings are validated during my follow-up appointment a few weeks after my last infusion. I embrace my new post-chemo independence and assure my parents there's no need for them to come in. I even let Missy off the hook. I meet with the physician assistant Sara who has been so supportive over the last six months. She greets me with her usual warmth. She always complimented my chemo couture. I admittedly did master the scarf as the perfect accessory. She is happy to report I am officially "free from evidence of disease."

I'm confused. "What about remission?" I ask. That's what they say in the movies.

"That's a term that isn't relevant to your cancer. This is the ideal diagnosis you want to hear. This is good news, Paige," Sara assures me.

I am entering the "survivorship" stage, which many women describe as the most difficult part of the journey. Sara speaks about the sense of loss that follows treatment and acknowledges that without the focus of the weekly treatments, my emotions have the freedom to finally express the trauma I have experienced physically and emotionally. She stresses the importance of different kinds of support (therapy, support groups, etc.). She explains that it could be up to two years before I reach the physical and mental stamina of my pre-cancer days. I learn lots of other overwhelming facts and emotional realities about this new phase of the journey and about Tamoxifen, which I'll start taking in a couple of months once I'm fully recovered from this last course of treatment.

I feel blindsided. Why didn't anyone tell me all this before? Tears well but I'm too tired for another breakdown. I say goodbye to Sara. I'll see her in a month at my next follow-up appointment. She gives me a hug, holding me for a few moments longer than I expect. Perhaps she anticipates the breakdown that is coming.

I go to my car and sit in the garage and cry, the same guttural cry from the Whole Foods Market parking lot over ten months ago. I feel completely defeated. The report of being free from evidence of disease doesn't even register. I can only see more hardship ahead. I pause and breathe. *In (natural pause) out. In (natural pause) out. In (natural pause) out.* My breath is always my best teacher. In a few moments I'm reminded of my recent realization about being present versus positive. It permeates my awareness. I close my eyes and ask aloud, "I don't know how to do this. Tell me how I do this."

My trusty sidekick, that small still voice, answers in a gentle whisper: *Let go of expectations, sweet girl. Be present and patient. Be kind to yourself. We are with you. You will be guided to take inspired action when it is time. Rest and nourish your precious body. Grieve what is ready to be released. It is OK to let go.*

"OK. Thank you," I say, somewhat confused, my eyes still closed.

We love you.

I open my eyes and look around. A wave of warm peacefulness washes over me. It's never occurred to me that I can converse with the still small voice. I feel her becoming more integrated in me. This is the moment I realize I am in mourning. Not just over the loss of who I was prior to my diagnosis, but also at the loss of the community I came to love and rely upon during treatment. I know enough by this point to embrace grief as a profound teacher, and welcome the lessons with an extra prayer for ease, grace, and compassion.

Chapter 16:

Purification

A COUPLE OF DAYS AFTER MY survivorship appointment, I show up at Flint's office. I'm weepy, raw, painfully vulnerable, and unsure of so much in my life. My guttural cries have become an ongoing flow of tears. Flint greets me warmly. He shares a personal reflection that when he feels in a similar state, it is like he is leaking.

Yes, exactly. Leaky tear syndrome—why is no one talking about this?

Flint reminds me that tears are one of the most potent indications of purification. Technically, it's a good sign that my body is in a regeneration cycle. *Like the butterfly,* I think. I'm amazed, as I so often am in my sessions with Flint, by his wisdom and technical expertise, and also that he shared a personal sentiment.

I report about my survivorship appointment and how blindsided I feel. I reluctantly share that as I emerge back into the world, I find myself wanting to let people know that I have survived cancer. I keep repeating, "I survived cancer" (while knocking on wood, because of my superstitious genes) almost as if I'm trying to convince and remind myself. I tell Flint I feel overwhelmed with the past and uncertain about my future. I'm paralyzed about moving forward. I share that I have not had the motivation to write, and that terrifies me because writing is my main line to my still small voice and the sacredness of this time.

"Flint, I feel grateful I got cancer." I can't believe I say it aloud. It feels confusing to confess something so morbid.

"Maybe you aren't writing what needs to be written, which I under-stand," Flint suggests. "To write now, in this emotional and uncertain state, requires an elevated vulnerability. But writing from this place is where you'll crystallize not just what you overcame, but the gifts you've discovered," he gently challenges. "The world that you've fallen in love with is an odd and unexpected blessing from cancer. Writing is where you'll be able to capture what you don't want to lose and what you want to maintain without illness as the prompt."

He's right. He's always right.

Flint guides me through a celebratory meditation to honor the road I've traveled to get here.

Use your breath as a touchstone to deepen your sense of body-centered relaxation. As you quiet your body and move into this space, recognize a fullness and ease that is a result of the good work you have done. This is not an invitation to let go of everything you've learned, but rather an indication you've done a really great job. That's something to celebrate. Appreciate how your diligent efforts and practice have supported your heal-ing journey. As you enter this interim period, know that what you have learned and these important aspects of self-care are essential to maintain. Meditation, relaxation, visualization, the ways you monitor and manage your energy to be gentle with yourself. Your healthy diet and exercise. The ways you've man-aged challenging work stresses. It's important to recognize what you've done so far because you've done a really good job.

With that appreciation, imagine moving to your reconstruc-tion surgery with confidence in your surgeon and surgical team and a beautiful result. You will recover quickly and without com-plication. Imagine what it will feel like to get the reconstruction, to regain a sense of balance, of proportion and fullness. That lovely sense of moving on and forward. This is a new foundation you've discovered. The things you've done maintain this healthy balance. Imagine a time when your body is not your primary focus. The wounds will heal. Your body will move beyond the treatments. You'll feel whole and robust again. Imagine what that is like in a healthy, joyful, active, and vibrant way as you see yourself fully recovered. You'll never lose the self-care. You don't do it because you're sick. You do it as a way of life.

Once again, celebrate how far you've come. Open to the possibilities of new life and the new ways you're engaging with life. Open to opportunities, most of which you can't see at this point. Imagine the loving and caring relationships that keep you in the heart of love that is the primary source of everything that fuels healing, happiness, fullness, and vitality. You are surrounded by it, held by it. It flows out of you. It is the energy that you are bathed in and that helps you heal. It extends to your family so they feel this healing and completion even as they embrace the newness of Paige. It's a more loving, open, and free version of yourself that this challenging time has helped you to realize. The path has been difficult, the gifts positive. So you keep the endless cycle of loving energy that opens you to nourishment. Always offer yourself gratitude for the time taken.

Flint closes the meditation. "Your journey thus far has been truly remarkable Paige; you need to know that."

I do. I do. I do be do.

Weeks pass, and I get to know the limits and capacity of my body. I take Flint's advice to consider self-care as something to incorporate into my life apart from cancer. I've always been a big proponent of self-care and frankly, I'm pretty good at it. Even before being diagnosed with cancer, I preached the important distinction between selfish and self-full, when we do things for ourselves.

I start spending more time with friends, taking on more work, and trying to introduce more movement in my life. I'm quickly fatigued but I note a subtle increase in my energy level with each successive day. *Win.*

My hair comes in as subtle peach fuzz. It's not the chia pet image I envisioned, but I'm grateful. My eyebrows and lashes grow back, probably at a rate of one per day. It's frustrating, but again, I turn to gratitude as my guide. Instead of attending the rigorous hot yoga class of my before-cancer days, I take cool, short walks in the crisp fall air, feeling my strength and stamina gaining.

The lessons of being present and patient continue. I let my body set the pace and nourish my body, mind, and spirit. I'm guided and protected daily by the still small voice within me. Kindness and gratitude remain absolute non-negotiables. It's starting to become very clear that these lessons aren't about chemo or cancer; they're about life. I'm a survivor now, learning to thrive. I'm reminded every day of the blessing I've been given.

Despite all of my soulful awareness, I still feel like I should be doing something more. My "doer" voice is antsy. It doesn't like any of the suggestions I'm getting from others, like attending a support group. I just don't feel ready. Courtney is amazing, but I am suddenly aware that she is further down the road, so I'm sensitive to not oversharing my frustrations with her.

My friend Jen introduces me to a book, *Second Firsts,* by Christina Rasmussan. Christina shares her journey of honoring the cycle of grief as a young widow and mother of two small girls. She talks about the "waiting room," where we sit in between our old selves and our new world order. It's safe in the waiting room and kind of hard to leave. Let's just say my waiting room is super cozy, so I totally relate as I read. I finally feel like someone gets what I'm going through.

Christina is scheduled to speak at my local bookstore, so I take myself out to hear her for one of my first evening outings. Jen was supposed to meet me but had to cancel at the last minute. Normally that would give me the perfect excuse to bail, but I'm feeling propelled by a greater force. I suspect it's my still small voice.

When I show up at the bookstore, there's a small crowd. There's no avoiding being seen so I take a seat in the front row. Christina shares her story of loss and the amazing transformation she has experienced by having the courage to honor the grieving process and re-engage with life in a conscious and loving way. I'm inspired, hopeful that perhaps the best is yet to come.

As Christina talks, I'm able to glimpse beyond the window of my own waiting room and see a future where I am living a life of love, vitality, light, grace, ease, mindfulness, creativity, joy, and laughter. I can envision all the things that I discovered at such a monumental level throughout my treatment manifesting in this future life but without illness as the catalyst. I also realize that while I am now technically deemed a survivor, my survivor self has served its purpose of protection. I can let her go. With her release, I feel the tickle of my new regenerating cells percolating with light. They shine as they break through into the world. I feel like I just took part in some sacred spiritual initiation.

The challenge is having the courage to open the door into this new life and all the uncertainty that it holds. But if there's one thing that this chrysalis of time has taught me it's that I can do uncertainty. Or rather, I can *live* with uncertainty. Staying present in the uncertainty provides the space so we can discover things about ourselves that we never knew and live from that place of faith and grace. For me and my still small voice, that's the adventure we were born to take part in.

Christina signs my book and we speak for a few moments. She looks straight at me and says, "I see that sparkle in your eye. You have unbelievable gifts waiting for you and a beautiful life ahead that you can't even imagine." I am overcome by her empathy and validation.

Most important, I believe her.

Chapter 17:
Reconstruction

A FEW MORE WEEKS PASS and it is almost the holidays. Earlier in the year, my extended family planned a trip to Mexico to celebrate Uncle Tim's 60th birthday. I was just starting chemo and wasn't sure whether I would be able to make it. It felt important to have something to look forward to, so I booked a refundable ticket, just in case.

As the reality of the trip begins to take hold, I feel anxious. I'm still in such a raw and vulnerable state physically and emotionally. My doctor assures me it is safe, as long as I take precautions since my immune system is somewhat compromised. Beyond the physical angst lies a deep emotional anxiety. I'm still trying to process this "survivorship" period. I've been thinking so much about Tricia and Sandy lately. I wish things had turned out differently for them, that I could sit down with my aunts and share our survivorship woes over a cup of tea, or in Tricia's case, a glass of scotch.

During one of my meditations, I become aware of the heart-wrenching realization that while I have felt so connected to both of my dear aunts throughout this journey, this is where our paths diverge.

They died, and I am still living.

I am overcome with grief I don't know how to process. I feel guilty as I prepare to see my cousins. I cry and cry and cry. Fortunately I have my monthly appointment with Flint in a couple of days, so I sit with the nagging sensations of heartache, fear, and sadness. It's so unbearable. I can feel myself shutting down.

No, no, no—stay open, feel what you're feeling. Stay with it. You're safe and not alone, says the still small voice.

But it hurts too much. I don't know how to feel this without crumbling.

Stay present, sweet girl, fully and without judgment. There is so much love surrounding you. Feel it, feel us. Let yourself crumble. From this rubble we will help you resurrect. You are not alone. My still small voice rings with an urgency I haven't heard before. It feels like she's called in extra support of angels and spirit guides. It's like being enveloped in a warm, cozy energetic blanket, like the one I was hooked up to before my first surgery. Gentle waves of love and grace course through my body, reminding me to take pause and breathe. *In and out. In and out. In and out.*

I'm reminded of all the moments of discomfort and restlessness on my journey thus far, when it would have been so much easier to disengage from the challenging moment at hand. But through the guidance of that unseen force I was propelled forward. I am aware of the vulnerability of these moments that serve as the catalysts of my transformation, that place where fear, judgment, anxiety, and uncertainty transmute into love, acceptance, compassion, and faith. I reflect on moments when my ego, which appeared to control so much of my life before cancer, was pushed aside as my spirit and that still small voice began to make themselves known. I acknowledge how vulnerability became my new norm, and grace my trusted new confidant. The juxtaposition of love versus fear is apparent in everything I experience. I see how much of my life before my diagnosis I lived in fear, doing what I thought I "should" be doing. What I now know down to the deepest part of me is that actions don't matter if I am unable to embody the deep reservoir of unconditional love that is available in each of us.

The path from fear to love is our ultimate journey.

When I meet with Flint a few days later, I share my recent insights around Tricia and Sandy and the guilt I feel. Flint explains that this is a common phenomenon called "survivor guilt." It's common among survivors of traumatic events such as war, natural disasters, accidents, and acute or long-term illnesses. He's glad that I'm bringing it up. It takes courage to face.

"Are you open to doing something a bit unconventional?" He thinks it would be helpful for me to have a conversation with Tricia and Sandy using a therapeutic role-playing technique. He will facilitate the conversation, which he believes will help me realize that my suffering or dying is not an outcome my aunts would want. He asks me to sit in the chair next to where I normally sit, and talk to myself as if I am my aunts talking to me. He has me close my eyes and take a few deep breaths. Warmth washes through me. I feel the sweetest presence. I know it's Sandy.

"What does she want to say to you?" Flint prompts.

"I'm so sorry you've had to go through this. And I'm so proud of you. At least someone got some good use out of that book," she jokingly refers to the Bernie Siegel book. I hear her laugh. "Now take these lessons and this open-heartedness and LIVE YOUR LIFE."

I am simultaneously laughing and crying. I thank Aunt Sandy for coming and acknowledge that I hear her unequivocally. "I miss you so much."

I swear I can feel her gently caressing my forehead. I am in awe.

The energy shifts, and I start sobbing. Tricia is here. I miss her so much it hurts. I don't hear her say anything, but I sense her pride. I'm reminded of one of our last conversations when I visited her at MD Anderson and she told me not to be afraid, to live my life and express my truth. I sense her giving me her signature smile as she says in her

Southern accent, "I love you so much darlin'. You have much to be proud of and to celebrate. Let yourself do that."

I feel as if the three of us are sharing a huge energetic hug. And then I feel them leave. I am back in the room, back in the chair, back in my body. My tears have stopped. Calm and peacefulness radiate through me.

"Good job," Flint says. "That was very powerful. Do you feel you can move forward and start living your life?"

Yes. Unapologetically yes.

I can't logically make sense of how Tricia and Sandy came through, but my spirit/soul/still small voice knows not only did they come through, but I can also identify their presence and know without a doubt that they have been with me all along.

As the new year arrives, I focus on the next phase of my healing. Everything comes full circle when I go in for my reconstruction surgery almost exactly a year after my diagnosis. I feel especially reflective. Despite the pain, poking, prodding, and discomfort, this has been one of the most important years of my life. Difficult? Yes. Meaningful? Absolutely.

My old ways of intellectualizing and problem-solving simply don't work anymore. I need to keep feeling where I am versus seeking approval from others. It's a little disorienting, almost like I'm rewiring my way of being in the world. It seemed so natural and easy during my treatment phase, but as the realities of life creep back in, I understand that staying awake is a conscious choice I make in every moment.

I grow anxious to distill all of the lessons learned and insights gained before the year mark hits. I know this won't happen, because life doesn't work that way. We are always evolving. Regardless, I'm craving that full circle moment, the completion, the bookend, the

check mark. As the popular quote from *The Sound of Music* so elo-
quently states: "When God closes a door, He opens a window." I realize that with most endings, new beginnings are on the horizon.

As I drive to MD Anderson, I recall the butterfly I discovered a
year ago. In many ways I too am emerging from the chrysalis. Instead
of getting wings, I'm getting new boobs.

I find an odd sense of comfort when I arrive at MD Anderson and the
Rotary House for my reconstruction surgery. Mom, Dad, and I meet
with Administrative Services to confirm that my surgery, as well as
any follow-up surgeries that I may need, will be covered by insurance.
We are old pros in Cancerland at this point. We go to the Lantern Café
at the midpoint of the skybridge for lunch, where our favorite table
overlooking the courtyard is available.

It's nice to be here under more optimistic circumstances as I start
rebuilding my life and my boobs. We are all relaxed and ready. My
pre-op process for the reconstruction is a far cry from the cattle call of
my first surgery. The surgery takes place at the Breast Center surgical
suite, not in the main hospital. It is quiet, no crowds, and the décor is
lovely, all the way down to the reclining lounger chairs. A nurse calls
my name, and Mom and I head back. From his recliner Dad tells me
he will hold down the fort. "Let's round home base, sweetheart, and
bring it home."

Dad has grown well versed in sports metaphors. I knew my request
in my Team Woo-Woo email to avoid terminology around battling
and fighting my cancer would be a challenge for him. Dad spent his
early years in the army, and he's always been the captain of battle
metaphors. But he didn't waver at my request. I've been amazed by his
use of sailing, running, golf, and now baseball metaphors, throughout
my journey. I giggle and give him a hug goodbye.

I get settled in my gown, surgical socks, and warm blankets. Melissa, my plastic surgeon, comes in with her usual warmth and assurance. She's happy to share this part of the journey because she knows it will help me to feel more whole. I hold on to her every word. "OK, I'll see you in there. Enjoy your nap." She smiles and walks out.

The surgery goes smoothly and I only have to stay in recovery for a couple of hours. I'm surprised to see Missy when I wake up. Evidently there was some back-and-forth texting with my parents while I was in surgery prep. I had convinced Missy that she didn't need to be here for the surgery. She's more than served her time in the caretaking role and the hospital is not her favorite place. (Not everyone shares my enthusiasm for Cancerland.) But Mom felt as if she was coming down with the flu and needed Missy to drive me home. The stress is likely overwhelming her system and her body is telling her she needs to rest. I know that state all too well.

While the role of caretaker is often driven by love, there is also an unspeakable sense of obligation and responsibility that is both sacred and unfair. My cancer journey has had a major impact on all of my family. I may never fully comprehend the ripple effect on their lives, individually and collectively. I think that's why I wanted to ensure they were all getting support in that first Team Woo-Woo email. I now understand the blessings that challenge can bring, and trust my loved ones' capacity to receive their own lessons in the timing that makes sense for them.

The days following my reconstruction surgery go pretty well. I'm so relieved to not have drains that putting ointment on the incisions doesn't faze me. I'm so accustomed to the stiffness of the saline expanders that the lightness and malleability of the silicone implants is a welcome surprise. I still don't have any sensation, but my boobs look and feel fantastic—like the real deal! This is validated in the coming days when several friends come to visit. I unabashedly introduce those who are curious to the "girls." I've become so adept at stripping in doctors' offices that the once modest self of my college days has transmuted into a boob flasher, ready to show anyone who asks.

"Feel them, they're amazing." I have to remind myself that this isn't always appropriate, especially with my male friends and my friends' husbands. I recall that moment with Courtney in my hotel room before my cousin's wedding. Now I get it. It's proof that I'm not broken, and I want everyone to know.

Chapter 18:
New Normal

A WEEK LATER IT'S VALENTINE'S DAY—my cancerversary. While my recovery is going great, I'm still moving a little slow. I don't quite have a celebration in me, but I want to honor the day, and plan to see Romy. While the "girls" are here, I'm still not quite ready for my final close up but am eager to catch up with my friend. As I walk up the stairs to her converted office/living room, I'm met by two 20" x 24" framed images of me that take my breath away.

The first image was taken during our first photo shoot, the day before I left for MD Anderson for my mastectomy. I look frozen. I had just returned from my cousin's wedding, and I remember feeling a strange mix of exhaustion, serenity, and panic. I am in awe at how Romy captured all of my worry and confusion. I was in uncertain territory, prognosis unknown. Ironically, my hair was the longest it had been since my college days. I don't recognize that girl. I feel sad at the stress and unhappiness on her features.

The second image lights me up. It was taken the day after chemo, when the steroids were still in my system and I was full of energy, almost giddy. I was stripping down physically and emotionally, discovering an authenticity in my spirit that felt so innocent, tender, and joyful. I remember feeling awake for what felt like the first time in my life. It's as if the still small voice has embodied my essence and is looking through me with pride, grace, and love. I don't even see the

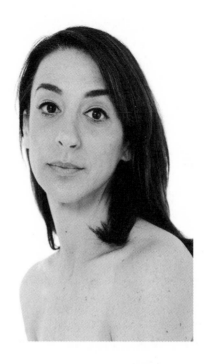

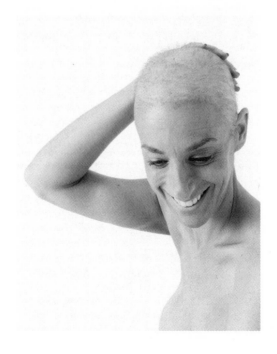

cancer. I look at that picture and know: that's the moment I started to fall in love with myself.

"Thank you, thank you," I keep repeating.

"Thank *you*," Romy says. I can tell this experience means as much for her as it does for me.

Back home, I place the pictures on my sofa. I can't stop looking at that second picture as I reflect on how far I've come in the past year. As grateful as I am for my year with cancer, I'm even more grateful this chapter has come to a close. I could not have done it without the unbelievable support of my family, friends, and co-workers. Now I can enjoy the blessings of that year without cancer as the catalyst. I'm proud of who I have become. I recall a quote by one of my favorite inspiring teachers, Kris Carr, a fellow thriver also diagnosed on Valentine's Day. "Curing takes place on the physical. Healing takes place on the spiritual."

I'm pretty good at this healing thing. It is integral to my way of being. Healing requires a willingness to love ourselves regardless of circumstance. In many ways, it is fitting that my cancerversary falls on Valentine's Day, for it marks the ultimate love story. I've fallen head over heels with myself.

Weeks pass and I get stronger every day. The upside to being so broken down is that moments of feeling good help me experience an entirely new level of appreciation. My taste buds come back and I enjoy food again. I'm using hair gel to style my new almost pixie cut hair. I look like a teenage boy, but I'm so thrilled to have something on my head, I don't care. I even start to emerge more socially.

I attended an event where I ran into several people I hadn't seen in years. One woman complimented me on how good I looked. "Such a fun short haircut," she said.

"I'm just glad it came back," I giggled awkwardly. She looked puzzled and then asked what was new. I launched into a long, perhaps dramatic, explanation of how, after having had breast cancer, I wasn't sure exactly what lay ahead for me. She looked at me with a blank stare. She had no idea I had been dealing with cancer.

At the start of my journey, several people had explained that I would start to look at life as "before cancer" and "after cancer." While I empathized with their experience, I thought surely it wasn't that black and white. I vowed that cancer wouldn't define me. But the thing is, it does. As much as I like to believe I'm out of my cancer bubble, it's very much part of my daily life.

I still wake up every Thursday morning thinking it's chemo day. I still have the gnawing fear at every meal that a wave of nausea will occur. I rely on my pillbox every morning to keep track of my medications. I step out of the shower every day and see the scars on my body. I have overwhelming moments of emotion washing over me at the most unpredictable times. I still feel annoyed that despite not having any breast tissue, I have to perform breast exams—always with a knot in my stomach. I find myself conflicted, not wanting to think about the cancer at all, and then suddenly terrified I'll forget.

Then there are the doctors who are quick to remind that it is never really over. There are no recommended body scans or blood tests; the only indicator of the cancer coming back is symptom-based. An ache is no longer just an ache—it might be a harbinger of something much worse.

I am learning to navigate my relationship to stress. Not all stress is bad. It's how we perceive it that matters. There's no avoiding stress outright. The truth is, we are living in stressful times. I see it in friends and family members who are getting married and divorced, having babies and raising teenagers. Caring for loved ones, changing jobs, moving homes, and so many other experiences that can make us feel like our lives change in an instant. As uncomfortable as these transitions can be, they also present the opportunity to soften the edges of our souls and live with more love, forgiveness, compassion, and meaning.

Despite the paranoia, emotion, and disorientation, all the lessons learned are slowly but surely inching their way into my consciousness. I'm more lighthearted, more present and loving. I enjoy myself on an entirely new level. I'm navigating how to set new boundaries while being open to new possibilities, staying responsible to my current obligations, and staying present, loving, and honest with myself. I decide it might be time to look into support groups and connect with other survivors.

I feel ready to emerge from my cancer bubble and step into my "new normal." I keep hearing this term from other survivors and doctors. It describes the survivorship period of post-cancer life once the treatments are complete and one enters life with the surreal experience of cancer as something endured.

I'm not alone in creating a new normal. My entire family emerges in new ways: Missy and her family move into a new home, something she's wanted to do for years. Megan and her husband move to a new city for a dream job opportunity. Mom and Dad finally start planning the cruise they put on hold when they learned of my diagnosis.

Courtney is now teaching yoga. She came for a visit, along with the rest of my college crew (formerly known as The Rack), in between reconstruction surgeries. Our shared experience is something neither of us would wish for, but it has bonded us together in the most magical ways. Our Facebook post from that visit says it all: *Breast Friends Forever.*

My boyfriend and I make a few attempts to find our way back to each other. Ultimately we decide it's best to simply let each other go so we can both find the love and happiness we deserve and desire. I believe our foundation was too fragile to endure the hardship of my cancer. Our post-cancer connection simply wasn't the same as when we first met.

Even BlueAvocado is going through a transmutation. While I am no longer involved in the day-to-day, I continue to be the company's biggest fan and support the team and board in various capacities. Our most popular product, the (re)zip, represents the new brand for the company. The (re)zip family of products are designed to minimize the use of disposal baggies. With this rebranding effort, the hope is to bring a product focus that will provide sustainable growth.

Flint is also making some changes. He's scaling back on private therapy to focus more on speaking and teaching. He feels I will be fine without our sessions, and sadly I have to agree. Our relationship shifts and we meet for tea and lunch, just like real friends. Then we make it official—Facebook and Instagram. Now I receive his wisdom in my daily feed. In one of our last sessions he helps me come up with action steps I can take.

1. Find a support group that resonates (don't force it, be patient, the right group will show up).

2. Book a session with an intuitive healer/psychic (don't worry, it's not like she can say anything worse than what you've been through).

3. Feng shui, the fuck out of my house (my words, not Flint's). Feng Shui is an ancient Chinese art and body of knowledge that helps to balance the energies of a given space. I became certified to consult spaces several years ago.

We close our session with a guided lovingkindness meditation. He explains that lovingkindness, also called *Metta*, is a simple, heart-centered meditation technique with roots in Buddhism. Practiced around the world, Metta cultivates compassion for oneself and others. Compassion is the natural state of the heart and mind, which is motivated by cherishing other living beings, and wishes to release them from their suffering. In this meditation practice, you gather your attention to focus on a specific compassionate phrase that you repeat silently. Flint reminds me that it is important to not force warm and fuzzy feelings or to get rid of unpleasant or undesirable ones. Instead of expecting to feel a particular way or judging and analyzing what I feel, I'm to allow whatever happens just to happen, with a beginner's mind.

Allow yourself to get settled and find your center, a place you have come to know over this past year. Bring your heart awareness to someone you care about or anyone you feel love for or who has been good or inspiring to you. Silently and sincerely offer them lovingkindness by silently repeating the following phrases.

May your body be at ease.

May your heart be open.

May your mind be boundless.

May you be awakened and at peace.

Refocus your attention on your heart. Continue to breathe naturally. With the same sincerity, offer the same phrase of compassion to yourself.

May this body be at ease and healthy.

May this heart be open.

May this mind be boundless.

May this being be awakened and at peace.

Return your attention to your heart center and bring to mind someone who you believe is suffering or in need. Offer them the same lovingkindness.

May all bodies everywhere be at ease.

May all hearts in everyone be open.

May all minds in all persons be boundless.

May all beings everywhere be awakened and at peace.

And finally, bring your attention back to yourself with awareness of the deep connection you have to all of these beings. Extend your blessing to those in your home. Expand it to include your neighbors, and all living beings in your city, your country, on Earth. Offer the same lovingkindness.

May we all be at ease.

May all our hearts be open.

May all our minds be boundless.

May we all be awakened and free.

Chapter 19:
Moving Forward (Kind Of)

As SOON AS I PUT MY ACTION STEPS out in the universe, as always, it provides. I'm connected to several survivors who are friends of friends. I immediately hit it off with a woman named Debbie. She's also a recovering Type A personality who has transformed through cancer. We meet for coffee and share the logistical and spiritual challenges we've endured. Debbie is further along in the reconstruction process and provides sound perspective. I'm currently assessing my nipple strategy as the next step in reconstruction. She explains to me the various paths I can go with my nipples. I've heard this from my doctors but hearing Debbie speak it firsthand makes it digestible.

"There are basically two paths. The first is nipple reconstruction, which requires another surgery. They go in and pull skin from your hip or butt and actually build the nipples. Once that heals, you get the tattoos of your areolas. This is the path I took because they look and feel more real." I am in awe of Debbie's articulation of the nipple reconstruction process. I'm unprepared for this level of detail and don't have any questions.

"The second path, which is all the rage these days, is 3D tattooing, a technique that looks like the real deal. The upside is that you don't need another surgery, just a Valium maybe for the tattooing." She laughs. "Do you want to see?"

We go into the bathroom so she can show me her breasts, complete with nipples. They look fantastic. Nipple reconstruction looks legit. Only with another survivor can I shop for nipples.

In addition to my friendship with Debbie, I learn about a survivors' group sponsored by a local organization that offers free Kundalini yoga classes at a studio just a few minutes from my house. I don't know much about Kundalini yoga except that it's a bit on the alternative side, but since I'm in daily conversations with my still small voice, I decide to give it try. I show up at the studio, the same one where I used to sweat and power my way through a good Vinyasa flow. I've been told this class is a far cry from that. Thank goodness. I don't have it in me to power through anything.

When I walk into the room, there's a big gong at the front, and a few women who all look like me, with spikey hair that is cute but obviously new growth. I smile awkwardly and follow their lead, grab a blanket and a couple of bolsters to place on top of my yoga mat. I sit on the bolster and wait for the teacher to arrive. I close my eyes and start to breathe. *In and out. In and out.*

The teacher walks in, wearing all white from head to toe. She emanates compassion as she comes over and introduces herself. "I'm Kelly. I'm so glad you're here."

I note that she has the same name as my friend Kelly. *Win.* A few other women arrive. Some are completely bald, and it is obvious they are in the midst of chemo. Others have longer hair, an indicator that they are on the survivor road. Sadness washes over me. All of these women have endured similar circumstances to my own. Instead of fighting my tears, I let them gently fall. I already feel safe and comforted in this space, with these people.

Kelly introduces herself to the class as an eight-year cancer survivor who suffers from occasional lymphedema (numbness and swelling of the arm). She shares how Kundalini was a tremendous resource throughout her cancer journey and continues to be. She invites us to close our eyes and chant the opening prayer—*Ong Namo, Guru Dev*

Namo (I bow to the divine teacher within). I get a pit in my stomach at the thought of chanting, but when I close my eyes, the chant effortlessly flows out of me. It feels like I've discovered a main line to my still small voice. For the rest of the class we do exercises that focus on repetitive movements while reciting mantras, Sanskrit words that awaken energies in our bodies.

At the end of the hour, Kelly invites us to lie down in *savasana* while she plays the gong. The vibration reverberates through my body. A wave of warmth and peace washes over me. I am hooked.

After class, I spend a few moments speaking to some of the other women. We all share where we are in our journeys as we enjoy a Dixie cup of tea. I feel lucky that I've connected with these strangers who I know are about to become integral to my new normal.

Next on the list, I meet with the intuitive who has come highly recommended from a friend of my acupuncturist. As I pull up to a building in west Austin where the session is located, I'm struck by the irony that it is next door to the Pilates studio I used to own. It is also located in the same office building where I used to get Holographic Repatterning years ago. It feels good to be back in that "feel to heal" bubble.

I walk in the door and am struck by the scents of lavender and sage wafting through the room. Barbara, the intuitive, is a tall and beautiful woman with long flowing gray hair. I feel like I'm in the presence of a goddess. I take a seat facing her. She grabs my hands and closes her eyes and takes several deep breaths. I join her. *In and out. In and out.*

"You've been through a cancer journey, yes?"

"Yes," I respond, although given my new hair growth, it is somewhat obvious. She continues to breathe and then opens her eyes.

"Do you know what the cancer represents for you?"

"Why yes, I do actually," I respond smugly. "One of the first things

I did upon my diagnosis is look up the meaning in my Louise Hay book, so I know it is about a refusal to nourish the self, and the importance of—"

She stops me mid-sentence. "You haven't learned what you need to learn."

My heart stops. *Excuse me? What the fuck? Then what has this past year been about? I paused. I surrendered. I nourished. I suffered. I put boundaries in place. I discovered a love for myself and others. What do you mean, I haven't learned my lesson? Did I manifest cancer?*

I don't hear the rest of the reading. Like the good ole' pre-cancer me, I shut down. When the session is over, I am in shock. I grab the CD Barbara recorded and drive home. She encourages me to listen to it later. "It will make more sense once you have some time to reflect," she assures me. I leave the reading devastated. I feel like all the work of the past year was for nothing, and worse, that the cancer is festering, waiting to come back.

Later that evening, once my anger and emotion subside and I'm more grounded, I listen to the CD with a new perspective. Barbara helps me realize I have a lot of fears that I'm not yet willing to face— the cancer coming back, dying, cancer affecting other members of my family. That evening I sat with those fears, giving them the space to exist without trying to rationalize or justify them away. I know from my meditation training that fear is a sign that our attention is likely in the future where we don't have any control. The best thing we can do is come back to the present moment. As I have so many times before, I breathe and let fear dissipate with each breath. *In and out. In and out.*

As I do this, I'm able to acknowledge that cancer has been an amazing journey of transformation. I have shifted my consciousness from one of doing and searching, from a place of fear and angst, to one of being and arriving at a place of stillness, connection, and listening to the deepest part of my soul. There will always be fear of the unknown, but I am more grounded than I was before. I'm armed with a deeper conscious awareness and tools that are shifting how I live my life with more love, peace, equanimity, connection, and joy.

Did I manifest my cancer? I don't know. It doesn't really matter. What matters is that I treat my body with the respect it deserves. That I nourish my spirit with relationships and activities that are fulfilling and meaningful. That I express myself with truth and authenticity. That I keep my heart open. That I stay connected and present to life. I continue to stay open to exploring new ways of deepening this conscious awareness, and to knowing that the universe always has my back.

Spring fever takes on a new meaning in Austin because it coincides with the South by Southwest Interactive, Film and Music Festival. For two weeks the city transmutes into a haven of parties and music. From gas stations to venue halls, it is a mecca of innovation and creativity. My body and soul soak up every ounce of this new energy.

I come home one afternoon after visiting a friend who's in town for the festival and suddenly the vibrancy of the city's energy is sucked out of me. All I see when I look at my home is my mini-version of Cancerland. While the soft gray tones in my living room were intentional to set a neutral theme when I moved in, now all I see is the grayness of my day threes. I walk back into my office, which is filled with piles of papers and medical bills I haven't had the motivation to go through. When I move into my bedroom, it's a sad place of extra blankets and my Relax The Back pillow, which has served its time.

I can feel the transformation of the past year but all the energy I released is stuck in my home. I tap into my feng shui toolkit to transform my cancer-centric home into a new space that will set the stage for my best chance of stepping into my new normal.

First things first: cleanse the space. I pick up a bundle of sage at

Whole Foods Market. It is very important when smudging a room to open all doors and windows so that the energy can escape. I learned this the hard way during my rookie days of space clearing at a start-up I worked for in San Francisco. It was a garage office with no windows. On a random Friday, I was convinced I needed to clear out the energy to help a pending investment. My co-founders were meeting offsite all day, so I was surprised when they returned unexpectedly and walked into a haze of sage smoke that perhaps could be mistaken for pot. Lesson learned.

Over the next several days I purge old clothes, medical supplies, bills, papers, and scarves. I reorganize my closet and get rid of some of the clothes that don't feel representative of who I am anymore—like the Ann Taylor suit I haven't worn in ten years. I decide I want to infuse my home inside and out with more vitality. In feng shui terms this means bringing in more fire elements of reds and oranges. I end up perhaps over-purging and suddenly find my home very open and spacious. There's lots and lots of space.

The emptiness feels uncomfortable. I want to fill it ASAP and peruse online shopping websites looking for the perfect accessories. But if there's anything I've learned through my cancer journey it's that if I can sit in the discomfort and invite a little surrender, the right thing, person, or circumstance will show up exactly when I need it.

Sure enough, a few weeks later I'm running errands when I stumble upon this random store next to the pet store where I go all the time for Buck. I've never noticed it before. As I'm walking by, I spy a metal peacock. It is big, heavy, bright, and clunky. Not at all my aesthetic, it stops me in my tracks, and I think to myself, *I have to have that*. I try to disregard it because it's pretty tacky. I proceed with my errands, but I can't get that peacock out of my head. I return to the store and buy it, with no idea where it will go. Technically it's described as yard art (I don't have a yard), but I recognize my still small voice and am learning to listen.

Curious as to what the deeper meaning is, I google "spiritual significance of a peacock." In many ancient traditions, the peacock is thought to have the power of resurrection, symbolizing renewal and immortality. It is also described as being a symbol of integrity and beauty if we endeavor to express and show our true colors. That seems pretty spot on. It's the ideal embodiment of where I feel emotionally, physically, and spiritually. Every time I pull up in front of my home or Buck pees on that peacock, I'm reminded to let my true colors shine through and to be kind to myself as I continue to reinvent my reality.

Instead of seeing these things as random, I'm choosing to embrace these little signs, however silly or insignificant they may seem, as virtual high fives from the universe reminding me that I'm never alone. And that circumstances, people, and random objects show up to remind us what we need to know in the moment.

Jews don't get tattoos. Whether fact or fiction, it was a Jewish rule ingrained in my psyche at a young age. Which makes it all the more ironic that about three months after my purging and peacock adventure, I find myself in the waiting room on Yom Kippur at age thirty-nine about to get not one, but two tattoos.

Instead of one of the hip studios on Sixth Street in downtown Austin, I'm in a sterile surgical room at MD Anderson. I know the drill: check vitals, rate pain, get naked from the top up, and put on a cozy robe.

For many breast cancer survivors reconstruction, specifically nipple tattooing, is the last step on the surgical journey. Many women are so tired at this point that they simply opt out, at peace with living a nipple-less existence. My own expectation is that this will be the easiest part. Technically it *is* the smallest. But the reconstruction surgeries are some of the most difficult physically, emotionally, and spiritually of my whole cancer experience. I had to have an unplanned surgery to fix my left implant. My doctor recommended we go ahead with the nipple reconstruction at that time since I would already be under anesthesia. While I had Debbie's experience as reference, I was unprepared in terms of my usual due diligence. I decided to go for it so I could have it behind me.

I wasn't prepared for the post-op reality of nipple reconstruction surgery, which left me with what looked like two phalanges sticking out of my silicone breasts. Melissa tried to warn me they would be swollen and large, but this, what looked like thumbs protruding from my chest, I was not expecting. Thankfully the swelling went down and now I'm thrilled.

The reconstruction phase took me by surprise. I thought completing chemo would be the bookend and launch me into the post-cancer "new normal" I had heard so much about. It was naïve of me, I realize now, but I didn't anticipate that ultimately Humpty Dumpty had to be put back together again and that would take an additional year of surgeries and recovery.

My doctor Melissa comes in. I give her a hug. "Wow, you look great!" she says. It's surreal to be here with her. I remember meeting her for the first time a year and a half ago, and her saying, "I will be with you until the very end."

The nurse practitioner/tattoo artist arrives. "Are you excited?" she asks.

"I'm actually a little nervous," I respond.

"Oh, honey, this is the fun part." I appreciate her passion as she starts blending the many shades of nude-colored ink. We test different sizes and shapes. I feel cold and awkward as she paints on the various color combinations.

"Oh, this looks really nice," she says about a specific color combo. Pale pink buttons or tanned wide spheres; I don't really care. I just want it done.

I sit in the chair with the needle pricking me for four hours. I'm not in any pain since I don't have feeling in my breasts, but as I hear the constant buzz of the needle, I relive all the random moments of my cancer journey: Valentine's Day, the day of my diagnosis. I still remember the look on my doctor's face as she reviewed my ultrasound.

Waking up from surgery still groggy and asking if it had spread. It had—they removed twenty-nine lymph nodes. The first day of chemo and that taste, that goddamn metallic taste. Sixteen treatments later, the last day of chemo.

When the needling procedure is finished, I feel physically complete (the nipples look fantastic). But emotionally and spiritually, I'm depleted. There's nothing more to hold out for, nothing more to stay strong for.

As I head to the airport, tears fill my eyes. The security line feels like it's moving slower than ever. I arrive at the gate, sit down, and check in with my family. All good, I tell them.

Then I lose it. Guttural cries at Gate 26B. Just like that first day in the Whole Foods Market parking lot. I can't hold on anymore. For some reason now, new nipples on, I can finally let go of all the fear and emotion of the last nineteen months.

No one sitting around me has any idea of what's just happened under my shirt, but I am met with the kindness of strangers. "Are you OK?" they ask.

The gate attendant comes over, puts her arm around me, and says, "Is there anything I can do for you?"

I take off my glasses and wipe my eyes. As she hands me a tissue I ask what every coach class passenger always wishes they could: "Can I pre-board?"

For many people, tattoos have a bigger, metaphorical significance. While I didn't go into the day looking for it, I realize my perky little tattoos do, too: the culmination of one stage of my journey and the embarking on another. It's a perfect full-circle moment—just like my brand-new areolas.

The captain comes on the speaker and tells the flight attendants to take their seats. As the plane soars through the air back to Austin, I recall the butterfly I discovered just days before my diagnosis. It finally emerged and took flight into its new beginning.

A version of this chapter was adapted from "The Surprising Use of Tattoos for Healing," OZY.com, 2/16/16.

Chapter 20:
Now What?

Dear Reader,

It's early on a crisp Tuesday morning in Austin, Valentine's Day, and my four-year cancerversary. I've just passed the infusion center where I spent most Thursdays for six months. I'm on my way to a studio just a few miles away where I teach meditation. That's right, I teach other people to breathe. In and out. In and out. Can you believe it?

"Oh Happy Day" is playing on my car stereo, a morning ritual I've started since writing this book, and I'm singing at the top of my lungs. A group of about fifteen handsome, athletic men on bicycles pull up next to me. I'm busted and crack up laughing. They laugh, too. And then I cry, because these are the moments that matter. The moments of heart-opening joy that can also be moments of heart-wrenching despair. It is the tapestry of these moments that make life meaningful; it's the dance of the dark and the light that illuminates our lives.

A few days ago I had my six-month check-in at MD Anderson. My health is good (knock on wood). I still don't have sensation on parts of the left side of my body but am gaining more mobility every day. I've had a few scares and scanxiety, which have resulted in more CT scans, MRIs and biopsies, but all have come back clear. There are things that must be monitored, but like every other visit prior, I leave with a bit more relief and lightness in my being. And of course a good cry.

As I was waiting for my appointment, the receptionist gave me a pager that would buzz when they were ready for me. I noticed the number on my pager was 2220. This was also the number of my hotel room. According to angel guru Doreen Virtue, "the most common way that angels communicate with humans is through the universal languages of numbers and music." 222 has to do with balance, manifesting miracles, and new auspicious and timely opportunities. Trust me, I googled it.

I continue to embrace these signs from the universe through the spiritual lens from which I'm living my new normal. I'm reminded of the quote by French philosopher, Pierre Teilhard de Chardin: "We are not human beings having a spiritual experience; we are spiritual beings having a human experience."

My still small voice and I are taking it day by day, with gratitude and compassion as guideposts. Peace is my new bottom line. Whenever possible, I choose to do things that fuel me from the inside out. My life is much simpler. I've started a new business where I work with individuals, companies, and teams looking to integrate mindfulness and meditation into their busy lives. It's not the same fast-paced entrepreneurial environment of my BlueAvocado days, but it's steady, fulfilling, and meaningful. I continue to nurture the love affair with myself, knowing this will nourish my relationships, too.

Which brings me to you, beloved reader. I offer my deepest heartfelt thank you. I trust this book landed in your life for a reason and I'm so grateful you chose to receive it. I had no idea that writing this book would actually be such a key healing modality in my cancer journey. Several friends and family members had concerns as I was writing this, thinking I was stuck in the past, unable to move forward. But having you in mind has pulled me forward and inspired a level of detail and catharsis that helped me to honor this unbelievable road traveled. Writing to you has helped me reclaim parts of myself I didn't even know were lost. It's helped me realize that cancer wasn't my crisis point, but rather a landing pad to seek meaning in my life and to step more fully into myself.

So thank you, thank you. I don't know where we go from here. But I know without question there is an energetic presence of love, healing, and protection all around us. This energetic awareness invites us to be present to the moments that matter, so that it doesn't take a catastrophe for us to wake up to our lives. It also makes us better equipped in the unforeseen times when the relationship, health, work, or personal crisis does show up.

There is no going back, no figuring out how to step forward, simply being in it with gentleness and non-judgment. This doesn't mean that challenging moments don't exist, but when they do, I'm much better equipped to meet them with responsiveness and self-compassion. It is this present-moment awareness that continues to be my greatest teacher. It's available to each and every one of us.

The pre-cancer me wants to top off my story with a pretty pink bow of an extravagant ending, where we can wrap up my cancer journey and send it on its way. But life doesn't work that way, does it? We're never really done. The divine experiences of our lives, whether through struggle or joy, keep propelling us forward on our journey to greater self-awareness and consciousness.

What I can offer is an update to the guidelines I set forth in my original Team Woo-Woo email. Only this time I share from a place of reflection and to remind me of the lessons learned. I write this from the perspective of my still small voice, who seems to be calling the shots more and more as I welcome her presence in every awakened moment possible. We all have a still small voice inside us, which actually isn't so small. Some may call it intuition, grace, or even God. It doesn't always show up as a voice, but rather a knowing, a feeling, a sensation, a song on the radio, being in nature, a call from someone we were just thinking about, and occasionally triple digits. At times things may seem messy, chaotic, scary, and with no real purpose. But I know I will always be guided into authentic alignment with the truth that will serve me and those around me to collectively heal and honor a way of being that honors the darkness as much as the light. May we each continue to shine brightly with this collective recognition.

With abundant love and gratitude.

Happy Valentine's Day!

Here we grow,

~Paige

Team Woo-Woo Lessons Learned

1. Stay open—this is still a love journey. We have a choice in every moment to recognize if we are in a state of expansion or contraction. Whenever I feel stuck or unsure of something, I always ask myself—is my heart open or closed? When I keep leaning into the expansion I find all I need in that space, even if it doesn't always feel so good.

2. Meditate—every day. Meditation isn't about doing it for the sake of doing it, but because it's daily exercise to connect our body, mind, and spirit. With a daily commitment we are shifting the landscapes of our brain so we can be more responsive and less reactive. We feel more connected to ourselves and others.

We are able to trust our intuition as we navigate the inevitable unexpected moments that arise in our lives. The greatest blessings show up even when we don't know we need them.

3. Express yourself—get to know your truth. Whether through art, music, writing, and a myriad of other outlets, our job is to tap into an expression that is unique to each of us. When I'm feeling stuck or unsure, I take it straight to my still small voice in Q&A style. I'll simply pose a question like, "What do I need to know?" The answers always come flowing through, maybe not immediately, but the guidance is always there. Our voices need to be heard even when it feels like people don't understand us. These expressions are a gateway to our most authentic selves.

4. Take pause—no more powering through. Physically my body won't allow me to go into autopilot—daily meditation practice is key to this. If things are starting to feel forced, I stop. I'm learning to be OK with the stillness and softness of the pause. It always fills me up in the ways I need. This doesn't mean I'm not a productive person, it just means I'm more mindful about where I'm spending my energy.

5. Connection is key—this is perhaps the most important lesson of this time, the realization that we aren't in it alone. It is our human condition to connect with others and to surround ourselves with people who inspire and support us. And of course we're NEVER alone in the universal sense. The universe ALWAYS has our back.

6. Lighten up—have fun. Create a joy list of all the things that fill your body, mind and spirit and tap into that whenever you feel like you're starting to take life too seriously. Keep this list handy—on your computer, your phone, your fridge, anywhere where you can be reminded that joy is calling. This can be as simple as hanging out with friends and family, drinking tea, watching a funny movie, walking your dog, or yes, singing and dancing to "Oh Happy Day."

7. Listen to your body—your body knows. Continue to nurture and nourish your precious body. Often the soul lessons that are waiting to be learned come through conceptually first and then ultimately need to be integrated and embodied. Yoga, walking, running, dancing, acupuncture, Pilates, massage, etc. Anything that keeps your energy in flow.

8. Celebrate the wins—bank that shit. It's so easy to remember the hardship or how things don't always work in our favor. But by recognizing these universal moments that often show up in the form of "coincidences," we strengthen the connection to the guidance that is always with us. Whenever you're lost or scared, simply ask for help, a sign—any sign. That still small voice (or however you wish to define this presence) will always find us in moments of surrender.

Finally—always, ALWAYS remember to be kind to yourself.

And so it is.

Acknowledgments

To Mom and Dad, thank you for being with me every step of the way.

Dad, your discernment, perspective, and motivation provided clarity in the times I needed it.

Mom, thank you for showing up for every surgery and treatment and being available 24-7. Your nurturing presence, strength, and grace kept me going in the most vulnerable moments.

To Missy, unfortunately I feel this journey was equally yours. Thank you for being my rock. I will never fully comprehend the spiritual ripple effect this has had on you, but I am so grateful for you.

Mark, thank you for being a steady and supportive presence throughout.

Eli and Ruby, thank you for bringing such joy and light to my life and for taking such good care of Buck.

To Megan, you dropped everything at a moment's notice when I asked, and provided medical perspective in the not-so-glamorous times. Thank you for being my big sister.

Steve, thank you for sharing Megan in the early days of your newlywed bliss. And thank you both for the steady flow of New York bagels that arrived on my doorstep.

To my aunts, uncles, cousins, second cousins, and entire extended family, thank you for inspiring me and keeping me going. I love you all.

To my teacher Flint Sparks, our serendipitous meeting was the compass to guide my journey. I'm so grateful to call you my teacher, mentor, and friend.

To my teacher Sarah McLean, thank you for making meditation accessible for so many.

To my medical team at MD Anderson, Texas Oncology, and my many alternative healthcare providers, thank you for always giving me space to ask my many questions and addressing them through a collaborative approach. Jennifer, Abigail, Melissa, Debra, Sara, Mercy, Brian, Melissa L, Stacy, Stephanie, Susan, Deva, Zelie, and the many other guides and generous spirits who continue to provide support.

To the many teachers whom I have never personally met but have been guiding forces in my life, your books will have a permanent home on my bookshelf. I hope one day to meet you in person: Oprah, Bernie Siegel, Deepak Chopra, DavidJi, Louise Hay, Wayne Dyer, Andrew Weil, Eckhart Tolle, Dalai Lama, Caroline Myss, Elizabeth Gilbert, Panache Desai, Christiane Northrup, Sharon Salzberg, Tara Brach, Mark Nepo, Christina Rasmussen, Doreen Virtue, Kris Carr, Danielle LaPorte, and so many more.

To my breast friend Courtney, thank you for mentoring and inspiring me on this journey. We are forever bonded.

To my extended college, high school, and San Fran tribe, Ivy, Ellen, Danielle, Sarah, Joanna, Carly, Timi, Meredith, Apryl, Elizabeth, Tina, Jamie, Regan, Rachel, thank you for your texts, calls, gifts, and visits. Your trips gave me something to look forward to.

To my Austin tribe, you stuck with me through the celebratory milestones and motivated me in the times I needed it. Kelly, Katie, Romy, Jen, Natalie, Maggie, Jane, Dan, Dave, Ben, Malia, Debbie, Amy, Kristin, Sunni, Morgan, Jig, Margaret, and so many others.

To my BlueAvocado family, thank you for your support and commitment to keep things going.

To the un-nameable many who were praying for me, your prayers, texts, well wishes, and "likes" were and continue to be well received.

To my publishers, Brooke and Lauren at She Writes Press, and my publicists, Crystal and Madison at Booksparks. Thank you for empowering my publishing path with such support, guidance, and collaboration.

To my editor, Bridget Boland, your guidance and encouragement to embody this book as a true spiritual expression has provided a confidence and appreciation of the craft of writing in new and inspiring ways.

To the many survivors and thrivers I have met, there is no one-size-fits-all when it comes to how one approaches cancer. I've learned so much from you all.

To the many precious souls whose cancer journey ended differently than my own, your presence and love is not lost. It lives in the hearts of your loved ones.

About the Author

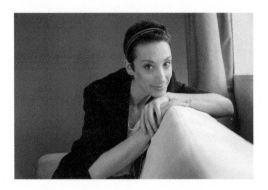

Paige Davis is an entrepreneur, writer, cancer survivor, mindfulness facilitator, and meditation teacher. She is the founder of Soul Sparks (soulsparks.com), where she leads and facilitates meditation and mindfulness programming for companies, teams, and individuals seeking more patience, productivity, and peace. Paige is a contributor to the cancer anthology *I Am with You: Love Letters to Cancer Patients* (Bay Tree Publishing, 2015). Her work has been featured in the *Huffington Post* and MindBodyGreen. She currently lives in Austin, Texas.

Websites:
www.hellopaigedavis.com
www.soulsparks.com

Social Media:
Instagram: @hellopaigedavis
Facebook: @hellopaigedavis
Twitter: @hellopaigedavis
Hashtags: #herewegrow
#hellopaigedavis

SELECTED TITLES FROM SHE WRITES PRESS

She Writes Press is an independent publishing company
founded to serve women writers everywhere.
Visit us at www.shewritespress.com.

Body 2.0: Finding My Edge Through Loss and Mastectomy by Krista Hammerbacher Haapala. 9781631521317, 16.95
An authentic, inspiring guide to reframing adversity that provides a new perspective on preventative mastectomy, told through the lens of the author's personal experience.

Note to Self: A Seven-Step Path to Gratitude and Growth by Laurie Buchanan. $16.95, 978-1-63152-113-3.
Transforming intention into action, *Note to Self* equips you to shed your baggage, bridging the gap between where you are and where you want to be—body, mind, and spirit—and empowering you to step into joy-filled living *now!*

Think Better. Live Better. 5 Steps to Create the Life You Deserve by Francine Huss. $16.95, 978-1-938314-66-7.
With the help of this guide, readers will learn to cultivate more creative thoughts, realign their mindset, and gain a new perspective on life.

This Way Up: Seven Tools for Unleashing Your Creative Self and Transforming Your Life by Patti Clark. $16.95, 978-1-63152-028-0.
A story of healing for women who yearn to lead a fuller life, accompanied by a workbook designed to help readers work through personal challenges, discover new inspiration, and harness their creative power.

Falling Together: How to Find Balance, Joy, and Meaningful Change When Your Life Seems to be Falling Apart by Donna Cardillo. $16.95, 978-1-63152-077-8.
A funny, big-hearted self-help memoir that tackles divorce, caregiving, burnout, major illness, fears, and low self-esteem—and explores the renewal that comes when we are able to meet these challenges with courage.

The Clarity Effect: How Being More Present Can Transform Your Work and Life by Sarah Harvey Yao. $16.95, 978-1-63152-958-0.
A practical, strategy-filled guide for stressed professionals looking for clarity, strength, and joy in their work and home lives.